THE
WELL-FED
MICROBIOME
COOKBOOK

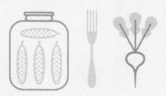

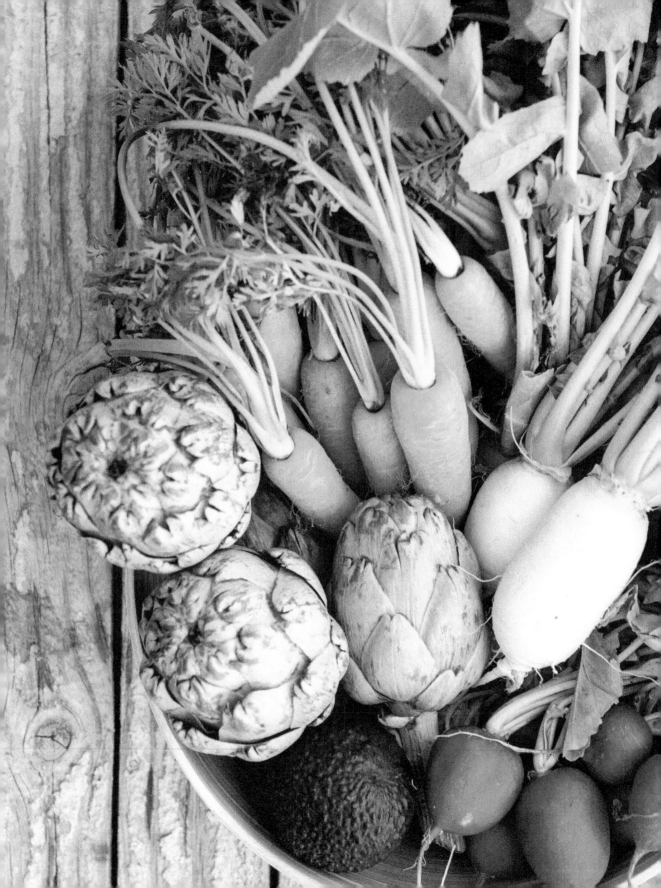

THE WELL-FED MICROBIOME COOKBOOK

Vital Microbiome Diet Recipes to
Repair and Renew the Body and Brain

KRISTINA CAMPBELL

**ROCKRIDGE
PRESS**

For general information on our other products and services or to obtain technical support, please contact our Customer Care Department within the U.S. at (866) 744-2665, or outside the U.S. at (510) 253-0500.

Rockridge Press publishes its books in a variety of electronic and print formats. Some content that appears in print may not be available in electronic books, and vice versa.

TRADEMARKS: Rockridge Press and the Rockridge Press logo are trademarks or registered trademarks of Callisto Media, Inc., and/or its affiliates, in the United States and other countries, and may not be used without written permission. All other trademarks are the property of their respective owners. Rockridge Press is not associated with any product or vendor mentioned in this book.

FRONT COVER PHOTO: Stockfood/Charlie Richards, Offset/Mark Weinberg.

INTERIOR CREDITS: Stocksy/Marta Muñoz-Calero Calderon, p.2; Stockfood/Maja Smend, p.6; Stocksy/Branislav Jovanović, p.8; Stockfood/Jalag/Julia Hoersch, p.16; Stockfood/Meike Bergmann, p.32; Stockfood/Danny Lerner, p.52; Stocksy/Nataša Mandić, p.70; Stockfood/Rua Castilho, p.72; Stockfood/Rua Castilho, p.96; Stockfood/Andrew Scrivani, p.120; Stockfood/Rua Castilho, p.146; Stockfood/Gareth Morgans, p.168; Stockfood/Gräfe & Unzer Verlag/Anke Schütz, p.220; Stockfood/Leigh Beisch, p.238; Stockfood/B.&.E.Dudzinski, p.262 All other photos Shutterstock.com.

ISBN: Print 978-1-62315-736-4 | eBook 978-1-62315-737-1

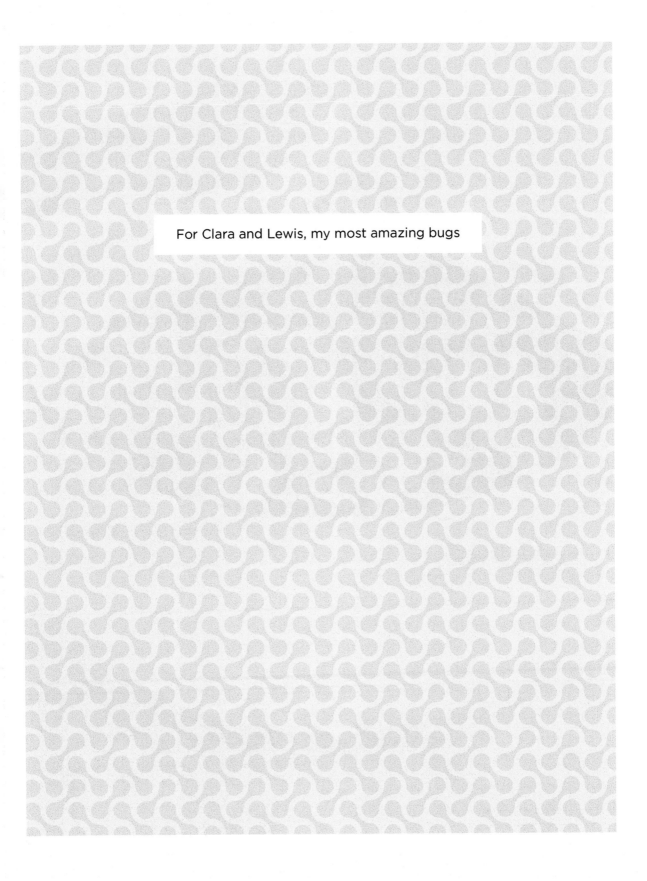

For Clara and Lewis, my most amazing bugs

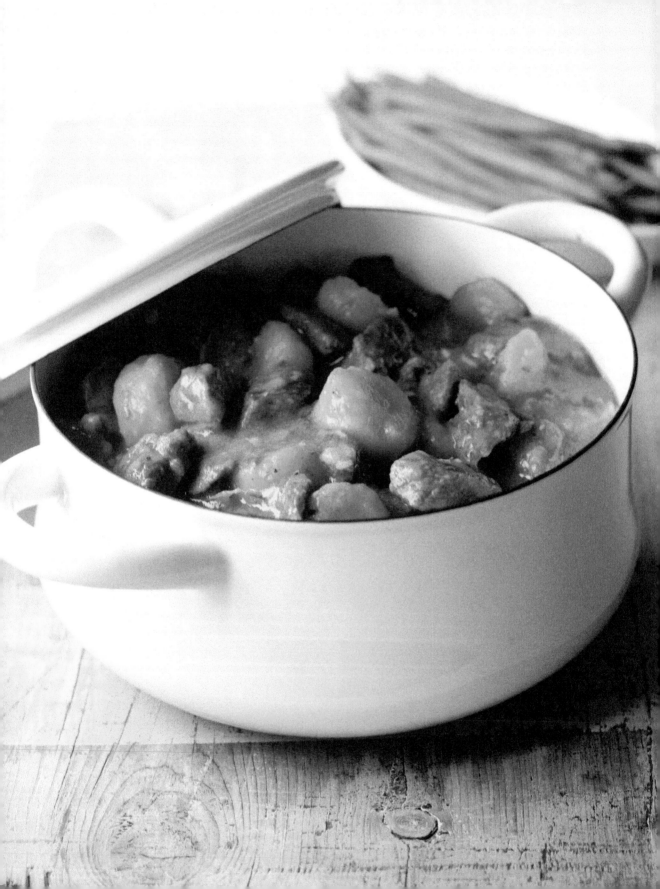

CONTENTS

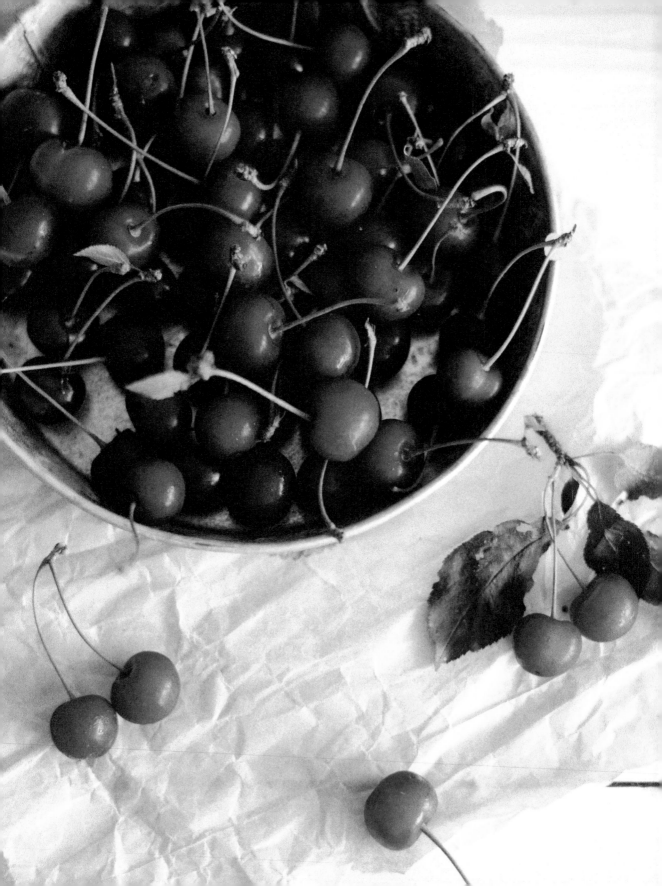

FOREWORD

ONE OF THE MOST PROFOUND REVELATIONS in biomedical research over the past decade is the critical importance of gut bacteria to our overall health. These microbes are redefining what it means to be human. We are not just a collection of human cells but, rather, a complex ecosystem comprised of human cells and microbes that, ideally, work together in harmony for our overall greater good.

The scientific understanding of our collection of bacteria, referred to as the *microbiota* or *microbiome*, is still, in many ways, in its infancy. However, with each scientific discovery in this area it becomes more evident that the bacteria in our gut are doing so much more than just helping us digest our last meal. These trillions of microbes are, in many ways, like puppeteers controlling the strings to our biology. They are intimately linked to the functioning of our immune system, wired into our body's metabolism, and closely connected to our central nervous system and brain. This is why many immunologists, cancer biologists, and neuroscientists are now taking a hard look at the power of the gut microbe.

While we still have much to learn about the complex ecosystem in our gut, over the past decade themes have emerged regarding how best to care for our microscopic companions. Our diet appears to be one of the biggest ways we can control our microbiota. Research from our laboratory at Stanford University School of Medicine, as well as other laboratories around the globe, have found that our gut microbes thrive on the dietary fiber found in plants, such as fruits, vegetables, whole grain, nuts, seeds, and legumes. Evidence is mounting that a diet rich in fiber promotes a more robust microbiota and reduces the risk for an array of modern chronic diseases, such as obesity, diabetes, allergies, and a number of autoimmune diseases. It is becoming clear that our modern Western diet—with its abundance of processed foods and dearth of fiber—has taken a toll on our guts and our health. The alarming rise in obesity, diabetes, and allergic diseases—not only in the adult population, but also among children—is a sobering wake-up call; we need to do a better job caring for our health or face an overwhelming burden of these diseases in generations to come.

As scientists studying the role of the microbiota in human disease, we are acutely aware of the dangers of an unhealthy microbiota. However, we have also witnessed the power of a healthy microbiota to treat and prevent disease. Our biggest hope, as scientists, is that our discoveries in the laboratory can be used practically to improve people's health and lives. Most people, though, don't have the time (or inclination) to weed through the scientific literature to figure out how to incorporate the latest scientific findings on the microbiota into our daily meals.

This is where the power of Kristina's book, *The Microbiome Cookbook & Diet Plans*, comes in. She has created an easy-to-follow road map that translates the exciting science on the microbiota into an actionable path to improve the state of your gut. Kristina's recipes include plenty of microbiota-promoting fiber, as well as fermented foods filled with beneficial probiotic bacteria. Her dishes are quick, easy to prepare, and taste good—all while keeping an eye on the prize, nurturing your gut microbiota. As working parents, we appreciate Kristina's effort to make her recipes weeknight-friendly and enjoyable by all members of the family. Our children are huge fans of Kristina's smoothies, and her Chocolate Chia Pudding (page 211) and Peanut Butter-Lentil Bars (page 216) have become staples in their school lunchboxes.

It is clear that knowledge of our gut inhabitants is revolutionizing the way we look at our health and will profoundly influence medical practices in the future. But until biomedicine can bring the promise of the research laboratory into the reality of your doctor's office, there is something we can all do to improve the state of our gut and, with it, our health. *Eating a fiber-rich diet* is one of the most powerful ways you can improve the state of this crucial community of microbes that live within, and rely on, us for shelter and sustenance. *The Microbiome Cookbook & Diet Plans* is really a cookbook for one of the most important things you feed—your gut bacteria.

—Justin Sonnenburg and Erica Sonnenburg, PhDs

Justin Sonnenburg, PhD, is an associate professor in the Department of Microbiology and Immunology at the Stanford University School of Medicine and received an NIH Director's New Innovator Award in 2009. Erica Sonnenburg, PhD, is a senior research scientist at the Stanford University School of Medicine in the Department of Microbiology and Immunology, where she studies the role of diet on the human intestinal microbiota. They are the founders of the Sonnenburg Lab at Stanford Medicine and the authors of *The Good Gut: Taking Control of Your Weight, Your Mood, and Your Long-Term Health*.

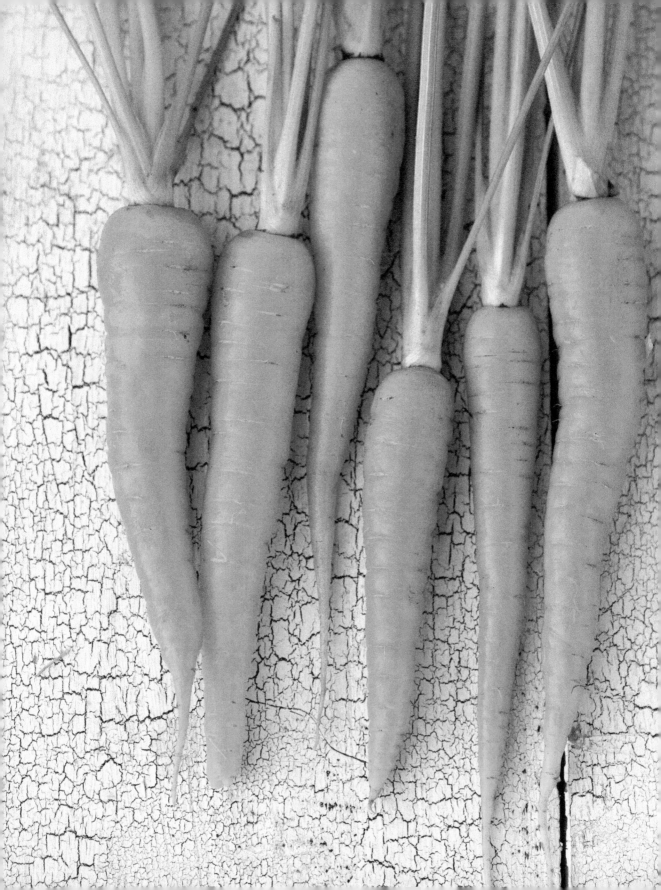

INTRODUCTION

I WAS RAISED IN THE COUNTRY, playing in the dirt of our organic garden. I ate spaghetti squash and beans almost daily. When I went to a university far from home, I shifted into cafeteria-food mode and didn't give much thought to my "freshman fifteen" weight gain and poor dietary habits.

My health decline was so gradual I didn't even realize it. I went from a healthy undergraduate to a young professional with some vexing health problems: skin rashes that came and went; constant gut pain and urgency; itchiness; brittle nails; never-ending exhaustion.

Then, one day, a jar of pickles in a cloudy-looking brine caught my eye at a kosher deli. They were a novelty—not made with vinegar like the pickles I ate, but with a simple salt brine—and I brought the jar home.

My first bite of a fermented pickle was different from anything I'd ever tasted. With the live lactic acid bacteria swarming on every inch, it was sparkling and alive on my tongue. It felt like a revelation. What was happening? I wanted to know more.

I bought a book on fermentation and found a whole new "culture" of food making. I wondered if diet could play a role in improving my health. From there, I got serious about "fixing" myself, asking doctors and experts for help and advice. I read news articles and popular books. I attended conferences and workshops. Through this long process I repeatedly saw compelling evidence of how diet affects the microbiome—the collection of bacteria and other micro-organisms naturally living in and on the human body.

I used my science background to dive deep into the research, and was aston-ished to learn nearly everything I did, from petting a dog to drinking a glass of wine, could affect the microbes in my digestive tract (or gut) that, in turn, affected my health. These microbes influence my weight, set the dial on my immune system, and affect my brain function. Fascinated, I devoted myself to learning more and, eventually, started writing about it professionally. I spoke with scientists in the fields of microbiology, pathology, immunology, and nutrition to find out what their work was about. Dozens told me they were troubled with claims in the general media that exaggerated what the evidence actually suggested. I resolved to be a translator for them, to provide reasonable interpretations of their studies for a wider audience.

I can tell you that most scientists now agree on one main point: diet can powerfully shape your gut microbiome and directly affect how you feel on a daily basis. Not all the hows and whys are clear yet, but the picture is filling in—study by study, piece by piece.

As a science writer, I have to caution that we need more evidence knowing precisely how each dietary change can steer our personal health. Patience is the only course. But as a parent, I need foods that will support my health and will give my children what they need to grow. Enter this book: the recipes here are based on information I've gleaned from the best studies on gut health available at this time. These pages bring together my two worlds.

To develop the dietary guidelines in this book, I carefully examined the studies that associate foods and dietary patterns with changes in the gut microbiome. I have presented the information in two parts, or phases. "Phase 1" draws from the body of scientific work concerned with alleviating symptoms of people not in the best of health. "Phase 2" is derived from the studies of people in general good health. This means whether you want to begin healing through your gut or you're in good health and want to maintain it, you'll find clear and simple guidance on how to take action.

Ultimately, this book is a collection of easy, affordable, and family-friendly recipes you can use to feed both you and your microbes. With tips on adapting recipes to your unique needs and a section on fermenting your own foods using inexpensive equipment, this book contains an abundance of resources for improving your gut health. I hope you're left with a good "gut feeling."

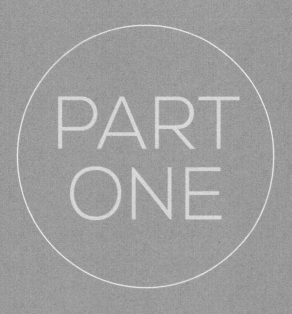

PART ONE

TAKE CONTROL WITH THE MICROBIOME DIET

We have an invisible "organ"—our gut microbiome. Science shows that the microbiome is integral to many of our bodies' activities, both in sickness and in health. In part 1 of this book, you will get to know your "intestinal garden" and why it's in your best interest to keep it thriving. You will also learn how to feed these trillions of microorganisms in ways that benefit you, the macroorganism.

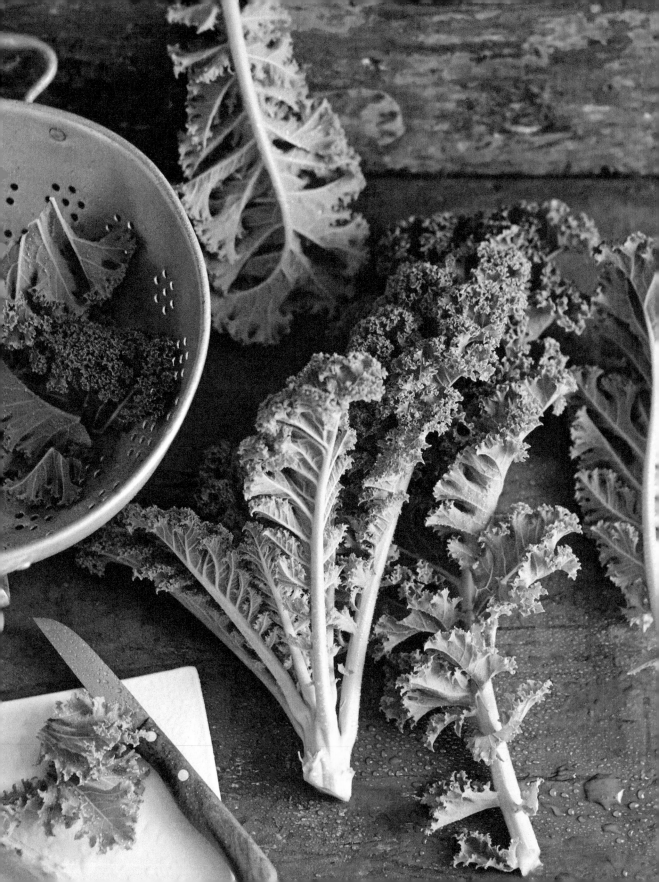

MEET YOUR
GUT MICROBIOME

With the help of science, we've learned that the traditional debate—
"nature" versus "nurture"—is not so simple. Your genes affect your
long-term health, of course, but there's another major player at work: your
gut microbiome. This community of microbes is both nature and nurture at
once, passed down from your parents (especially your mother) and also
influenced by environment (being extremely sensitive to what you do and
where you go). With diet, you can manipulate your gut microbiome. This
chapter explains your gut microbiome and how it can affect your health,
and it shares ways to nourish these vital bacteria.

YOUR INTESTINAL GARDEN

Many types of microorganisms exist as a living "varnish" over everything on the planet. They're in the water and air, on every grain of sand at the beach, on your pillow, in your food, and, of course, on the inside and outside of your body.

For decades, the study of these tiny organisms, led by pioneers such as Louis Pasteur and Robert Koch in the nineteenth century, progressed little by little. Research was slow and tedious, limited by the lab tools available. By focusing primarily on pathogens (disease-causing bacteria), scientists of the time cemented the common idea that bacteria were bad and harmful.

Advances in science and technology have changed the research game. In recent years it has become possible—and economical—for scientists to use DNA-sequencing technologies to take a "census" of the microorganisms (many of them harmless or even beneficial) present in any given place, opening their eyes to complex hidden worlds.

Your gut is a diverse neighborhood with hundreds of different bacterial species.

Different kinds of microorganisms live in different places. Some prefer the smooth surface of a light switch, while others like to hang out in your ear canal. "Microbiome" refers to a complete habitat that includes microorganisms (bacteria, but also viruses, archaea [a domain of single-celled microorganisms], and fungi), along with their genes and the surrounding environmental conditions. There is a second definition that refers specifically to the genes and genomes of the microorganisms in a given place, but we'll be using the first definition throughout this book.[1] Scientists are actively studying the microbiome of almost every imaginable nook and cranny: the microbiome of kittens, computer keyboards, gas pump handles, and of course, the human body.

While microbes cover every inch of the body and do important work in each habitat, your digestive tract—technically known as the "gut"—is control central. Microbes are at their densest concentration in your gut and many of the important jobs they do in your body begin there.

A Healthy Microbiome for a Healthy You

If you could peer inside a healthy colon, you would see a busy and thriving—but rather dystopian—community of microbes. Some bacteria jet around on little propellers (flagella), while others glide to and fro under their own power. They send out signals and bump into each other and sometimes have all-out wars, trying to kick each other out of the neighborhood. Some order the construction of factories that churn out a huge pile of products before being quickly dismantled. Viruses lurk. It's survival of the fittest. The dead are shipped off en masse every day, flushed out of the body and down the toilet.

Let's get this out of the way right now: in microbiome science, fecal samples are like gold. Used to find out what kinds of bacteria you're harboring in your gut, these samples are precious sources of data and are often stored for years in lab freezers. Different methods of sequencing the samples' DNA can tell scientists the different types of bacteria that live there.

You have a gut microbiome, like a fingerprint, that is uniquely yours.

If you compared a bar graph of the bacteria living in your gut with that of someone else, you would see huge differences. You would have more species in common with someone who lived in your household than with your neighbor down the street, and, in turn, you would show more similarity to your neighbor, gut-wise, than with someone living on another continent. Despite these differences, it would still be possible for all of you to be perfectly healthy.

In your gut, microbes normally serve the following functions:

- Making essential vitamins, including vitamin B_{12}, vitamin K, and folate
- Breaking down fiber you can't digest and producing short-chain fatty acid molecules that nourish the cells of your colon
- Protecting the gut wall to keep harmful substances out of the blood
- Defending against disease-causing microorganisms by out-competing them for resources
- Regulating your immune system and turning inflammation up or down
- Influencing the calories you harvest from food

From this list, it's easy to see how microbes could play an important role in how we feel. Indeed, scientists are finding out that the functioning of your gut ecosystem can affect your health in profound ways.

The question of what makes a properly functioning microbiome is not an easy one to answer, since the microbiome of a healthy person can look many different ways. One rule of thumb applies, however: A more diverse gut microbiome is associated with better health. If you house many different species of bacteria with different strengths and weaknesses, the microbes keep each other in check. A gut with many different species is less likely to descend into chaos when it

Both human genes and microbial genes influence your weight and your health.

encounters a threat from outside, or so the thinking goes. Scientists have found that many different diseases and conditions are characterized by a less-diverse gut microbiome.

THE LOWDOWN ON DYSBIOSIS

You want to aim for gut microbiome diversity because diversity creates balance and resilience. But if you took a look at the colorful graph illustrating the different bacterial groups in your gut microbiome, how would you know if it's diverse and balanced *enough*?

You might have heard the word *dysbiosis* to describe an imbalance in the gut microbiome. The word is often vaguely defined as a shift toward more pathogens or away from beneficial bacterial species. Some popular experts cite it as the underlying cause of a host of conditions, from bloating and fatigue to "brain fog."

In scientific studies, dysbiosis simply refers to some kind of difference. To cite one recent example, researchers from China found differences—or a dysbiosis—in the gut microbiomes of individuals with rheumatoid arthritis (RA) that distinguished them from a comparable group of healthy people.[2] In this context, the pattern found in those with RA may be called a dysbiosis because it is different from the gut microbiome of a healthy person and is associated with a clear disease state, even though the gut microbial profiles of those with RA were not so uniform that they could be used to diagnose the disease. So, in this study and hundreds more like it, dysbiosis is a general description, not a recipe or diagnosis.

A problem arises when trying to translate the concept of dysbiosis into medical practice. When it comes to individual patients, the idea has two fatal flaws:

1. **Dysbiosis does not map onto specific symptoms:** If you took two people with identical symptoms—say, bloating after eating the same foods—they might have very different-looking gut microbiomes; if you took two people with a similar profile of gut microbes, their symptoms might be totally different from each other. At this stage in what we know, your gut microbiome profile does not add anything concrete to what a doctor knows about you.

2. **Dysbiosis cannot be precisely defined:** Since microbes live in a complex community where they can substitute for and do each other's jobs, there is no definitive list of microbes that make up a dysbiotic microbiome. It depends. Too much of a so-called "bad" microbe might appear to be present, but perhaps

another microbe is keeping it from getting out of control. Dysbiosis could, therefore, take an almost infinite number of forms, so it is currently impossible to create a set of criteria against which to judge an individual sample.

Dysbiosis, then, is not an accepted medical condition. It can be more accurately defined as a gut microbiome difference associated with poorer health. Rather than trying to find out if you have dysbiosis, you would be better off starting with your physical symptoms and finding out whether scientists know anything about the gut microbiomes of people with those symptoms. With more time and more studies, researchers may learn enough specific information about the gut microbiome of each condition—like irritable bowel syndrome (IBS) or maybe even "brain fog"—that they could use it as a biomarker of that condition.

Factors that Diminish Gut Microbiome Health

While there is still a lot to learn, scientists have discovered some factors that can change the gut microbiome in ways that may be detrimental to health. These include:

Antibiotics: These powerful but overprescribed drugs change the gut ecosystem, sometimes permanently. Some kinds of antibiotics seem to be especially harmful when administered early in childhood.

Cesarean section births: Coming into the world is an important opportunity for a baby to be colonized by the microbes that set up their immune system for later in life. While a baby born vaginally acquires a gut microbiome from the microbes in the vagina, a baby born by cesarean section has a gut microbiome that more closely matches the one found on adult skin. These differences are being linked to the risk of asthma and allergies years later.

Overly hygienic lifestyles: Lack of exposure to a diverse collection of microbes is associated with poorer health—for example, a greater risk of allergy. Exposure to microbes from siblings, dogs, and rural environments help counter this problem.

Poor diet: Starting early in life, diet is important. Formula-fed infants have a gut microbiome that is less "protective" than that of breastfed infants. Later in life, dietary choices can reduce gut microbiome diversity and have negative effects on health.

Stress: In some young animals, stressful events can induce changes in the gut microbiome that last into adulthood. Researchers think that, in both animals and humans, the microbiome disruption caused by stress may result in different levels of activation in the immune system.

Infection: Sometimes when pathogens invade your gut, the intestinal ecosystem can really take a beating. Recent evidence from the US National Institutes of Health even suggests that certain infections can "scar" your immune system through their effects on the gut microbiome.[3]

While each factor on its own may not necessarily raze your gut microbial community or have obvious effects on your health, studies on the overall population have indicated, as a general pattern, that these factors are associated with poorer health and it's probably because of the ways they alter the gut microbiome.

THE DAMAGED GUT, WEIGHT, BLOOD SUGAR, AND MORE

All around the world, researchers have studied the guts of people with various conditions. From a mass of data generated in many places, from South American villages to urban Europe, they are zeroing in on a list of conditions that may have something to do with alterations in the gut microbiome.

It's not enough to discover that the gut microbiome of people with a certain diagnosis looks different from that of healthy people. Scientists never jump to conclusions—they know when two things occur together it doesn't always mean one causes the other. Think of it this way: we might observe a higher incidence of people wearing rubber boots when it rains, but it doesn't mean that rubber boots cause the rain. So, a distinct gut microbiome in someone suffering from ulcerative colitis (UC), for example, is worthy of notice, but it doesn't mean the gut microbiome caused the disease. It's merely a starting point for investigation.

To see whether a condition is actually caused by the gut microbiome, scientists have to look for other evidence. Microbiota transfer experiments are one such kind of evidence. Let's say researchers take two groups of mice: one group with a mouse version of UC (with its distinct gut microbiome) and another group raised in a sterile environment without any gut microbes at all. The scientists can transfer the gut microbes from the first group of mice into the second group, and if the second group of mice develops mouse UC, too, it could mean the microbes helped cause it.

Evidence from humans can also strengthen the case. Researchers might try to affect the gut microbiome of a person with UC by getting the person to consume a certain kind of probiotic bacteria. If the gut-changing intervention altered the course of the disease, it would be good evidence that the gut microbiome helped cause the disease in the first place.

Health Conditions Linked with a Damaged Gut Microbiome

With all this information in mind, the following list includes conditions that meet two criteria: first, scientists have observed a gut microbiome that is different from that of lean, healthy people, and second, evidence exists that microbes might play a role in causing the difference.

Obesity: In this complex condition, the intestinal microbiome may play a role in the metabolic changes and inflammatory processes that induce weight gain.

Diabetes: The gut microbiome has emerged as a key factor in the blood sugar dysregulation in type 2 diabetes.

Inflammatory bowel disease (IBD): Crohn's disease and ulcerative colitis are among the most widely studied diseases in the field of gut microbiome research. Scientists are starting to see that the gut microbiome plays some role in causing these diseases.

Allergies and asthma: New research links these conditions to how the gut microbiome "programs" the immune system early in life.

Irritable bowel syndrome (IBS): This is a functional disorder, based on reported symptoms rather than objective measurements. Studies of the intestinal bacteria of people with IBS are showing that it may indeed have biological markers and that it may have several subgroups that could one day be identified by gut microbiome analysis.

Colon cancer: Mostly attributable to environmental causes, this form of cancer has been linked to changes in the microbiota. The changes may happen when an individual consumes a diet too high in fat and too low in fiber.

More research is needed on other conditions, such as cardiovascular disease, childhood malnutrition, rheumatoid arthritis, nonalcoholic fatty liver disease, and chronic kidney disease. These are all associated with different gut microbiomes, but so far scientists cannot say with certainty that they are caused by

CRAVINGS: MY MICROBES MADE ME EAT IT

Cravings are understood as conditioned responses to cues in our environment. For example, we might not even think about a *pain au chocolat* until we see (and smell) a bakery shelf filled with fresh pastries, but, once we do, the desire to have one completely takes over our thoughts. Cravings can be so overwhelming they seem to come from forces outside our control. Is it possible that something else—like our gut microbiome—is trying to control our eating behavior?

A recent review in the journal *BioEssays* argued that since gut microbes rely on a human "host" for survival, they might, in theory, evolve ways to make us eat the nutrients that help them grow stronger, generating cravings.[4] This implies that microbes can act as parasites, causing us to behave like zombies, shoveling things into our mouths to please them. The paper laid out different ways this could happen: by directly affecting our behavior through communicating with the brain, by altering our taste receptors, or perhaps by triggering changes in appetite-related hormones.

So far there is little evidence to support this idea. The most relevant studies performed on rodents have shown that when certain benign gut bacteria are fed nutrients, their numbers grow rapidly until they start making particularly high amounts of a protein that acts like an appetite-curbing hormone.[5] In other words, the gut bacteria, through their protein messengers, stimulated hormones that told the mice they had eaten enough.

But helping orchestrate hormone release after eating is very different from hijacking your behavior and causing you to eat the food that microbes need for their own survival. Future research will determine how bacterial signals factor into hunger and cravings and how this fits into everything we already know about appetite control.

shifts in gut microbiome. (For more information on all of the conditions listed here, see gutmicrobiotaforhealth.com.)

In reading through the scientific literature, one might notice that many of the disorders listed previously could relate to inflammatory processes gone awry. Inflammation is part of how the body maintains and repairs itself, under the direction of the immune system. If the dial on the immune system is set too low (with reduced numbers of protective molecules being produced), harmful invading microbes may not be eliminated; if the responses are too high, the body may start damaging its own healthy tissues. In either case, the "fight" response—inflammation—occurs.

It is possible that unchecked inflammation could be a part of how some (or all) of the diseases on the list arise: Perhaps an alteration in gut microbes affects the immune system so it fails at its task of regulating inflammation, either in one specific location or throughout the body. If true, this would be an elegant explanation for the origin of many chronic illnesses. But the processes are complex and the science is at an early stage. Researchers don't know enough yet to confirm it one way or the other.

And now for the $920 million question: Is the gut microbiome responsible for the dramatic shift in the types of illnesses affecting humans in the past century? According to a 2016 report in *Nature Microbiology*, the United States alone spent $920 million on microbiome research to try to answer this question. Instead of contracting the feared infectious diseases of the past like polio and smallpox, people in the United States and other industrialized countries now suffer from conditions that affect their long-term quality of life—obesity, allergies, autoimmune diseases, digestive issues, and brain-related disorders, to name a few. Could this change be due to shifts in our microbiomes? In her book *10% Human*, science writer Alanna Collen explains in detail how successive generations have changed lifestyles—they've become more liberal with the use of antibiotics and more dependent on prepared and processed foods—while our microbiomes have been on a steady decline. So far it's not certain that changes to our microbiomes are driving these population-wide changes in health, but as researchers continue to investigate, they will get closer to the answer, condition by condition.

GUT FEELINGS AND THE MIND-BODY CONNECTION

The English language is full of metaphors like "gut feeling" and "butterflies in your stomach" that link the gut with the brain. Somehow the gut knows almost instantly when the brain experiences stress. This is because the brain and the digestive organs constantly communicate, sending messages back and forth— and it seems your friendly microbes, once again, are involved.

Spanning the distance between the gut and the brain is a path called the *vagus nerve*. It relays electric impulses along its fibers, between the colon and the brainstem with links to other parts of the body. Microbes can activate these nerve impulses, and this might be one important way they affect the human brain. So how much influence does the gut have on our mental and emotional health?

A smattering of evidence suggests that changing the gut bacteria can make a healthy person better at weathering the normal emotional ups and downs of daily life. In one famous study, University of California researchers gave women a fermented milk product (containing probiotics, or live bacteria) twice a day for four weeks.[6] They scanned the women's brains with functional magnetic resonance imaging (fMRI) and found the women showed positive changes in the brain regions that usually handle emotion and sensation. Another study by French researchers gave a probiotic supplement to study subjects and found "beneficial psychological effects."[7] And a different sort of study—one that tracked people's activities in daily life—found that young adults who consumed more fermented foods like miso and traditional sauerkraut, which typically contain live bacteria, experienced less social anxiety.[8] These studies all support the idea that modulating the gut microbiome with probiotic bacteria can help stabilize emotions in a general way.

The stakes get higher when we consider more serious challenges to brain health, such as depression. Researchers in China found that the gut microbiome of someone with depression is, on average, different from that of a person without the condition.[9] The bacterial communities in people with schizophrenia, autism, some forms of anxiety, Alzheimer's disease, Parkinson's disease, and severe alcohol dependence are all different from those in healthy individuals, too. By changing the microbiome, could we change the messages to the brain, thereby unlocking new treatments for these brain-related disorders?

Unfortunately, we have almost no data on changing the gut microbiome in people with these diagnosed conditions. This area of research will likely proceed more slowly than other areas, since mental health and emotional health are notoriously hard to study. You can measure cognition and emotion in many ways, from fMRI to questionnaires, but, because everyone's life is complicated, you can never capture every aspect of what people think and feel. Not only that, but we would need to conduct experiments with animals to show how the mechanisms work—and it's unlikely that a mouse's anxiety is exactly the same as a human's anxiety.

One provocative idea related to the gut-brain axis is that microbes can determine our personality. This may have some truth when it comes to animal models:

In 2011, Canadian researchers found that microbes can change a mouse from anxious and timid to brave and self-assured by affecting levels of a protein called brain-derived neurotropic factor.[10] In humans, however, it is likely more complex. An interesting development in this area is a study that found links between toddler behavior and gut microbiome profiles.[11] Children aged 18 to 27 months who were more extraverted had a greater diversity of bacteria in their guts; in boys, increased levels of particular bacteria were associated with traits like sociability. There could be many possible explanations for these links, though: it could be that toddlers who have more tantrums end up on the floor more often, picking up different bacteria that colonize their guts. Human studies on microbes and personality have a long way to go.

The gut and the brain communicate all the time. The task facing scientists is to delve deeper into the molecular actions that allow gut-brain communication to take place—and which actions are orchestrated by microbes—to help us understand the importance of this communication in human health.

FEEDING YOUR MICROBIOME

The basics of how you get energy from food are simple enough. Food has calories. You consume the food, and your body uses those calories. Consuming too many calories will cause weight gain.

The new twist is that your gut bacteria mediate the metabolism of your food. Feeding your ecosystem of microbes requires some special attention. You need to focus on feeding your gut microbiome for two reasons:

1. **Gut microbes act as a filter between the food you eat and the rest of your body:** A 2011 paper coauthored by leading microbiome scientist Jeffrey Gordon noted, "The nutritional value of food is influenced in part by the structure and operations of a consumer's gut microbial community."[12] This means that the number of calories you harvest from a given food depends on the bacteria living in your digestive tract.

2. **Your gut microbiome changes in response to your diet:** Within 24 hours of a dietary change, scientists can observe shifts in the gut microbial community. Certain components of the diet affect which microbes proliferate in the gut, as well as the molecules they produce. Some of these molecules, like short-chain fatty acids, are known to act at distant sites in the body and have major effects on your health.

Through diet, you can influence which individual species, or groups of species, thrive or die off in your gut microbiome. In essence, you can change the filter through which your food passes. But how does a change in diet shift the microbiome?

Certain parts of your diet are linked with the growth of certain bacterial groups. For example, *Prevotella* grow best when you have a diet rich in plant-based foods. The phylum (group) Bacteroidetes proliferates when certain fats are present. People in Japan even have healthy populations of specialist microbes that digest the seaweed in their diets.[13]

This seems simple at first: Feed each microbe its preferred food, and its numbers will grow. But no one actually knows yet if this is how diet changes the gut microbiome. You can't assume that if you eat more bacon, the bacon-loving microbes will proliferate. Maybe it's more complicated than that. Maybe if you eat more bacon, the immune system leaps into action and tells your body to compensate for the bacon's detrimental effects on health; the microbes that proliferate may not be the ones that love bacon but the ones that protect you from the fatty food. Furthermore, the gut microbiome's responses to diet could vary from person to person. There's much to explore.

Food can affect microbes, which "talk" to your immune system.

Despite these complexities, certain types of foods clearly benefit our microbiomes. Above all, you need to know about probiotics and prebiotics.

Probiotics, Prebiotics, and Synbiotics

Certain foods have a special status—a platinum card, if you will—when it comes to their ability to affect the gut microbiome positively. Two categories of food in particular, probiotics and prebiotics, have scientific support for their beneficial health effects.

Probiotics

The Food and Agriculture Organization of the United Nations and the World Health Organization define probiotics as "live microorganisms which, when administered in adequate amounts, confer a health benefit on the host." Every true probiotic, whether consumed in food form (as in commercial yogurt) or supplement form, must not only consist of a known bacterial strain or strains, but must also have adequate scientific evidence backing up its health effects. In mainstream media, however, the word *probiotic* is used widely to refer to any consumable bacteria, such as those that naturally occur in traditional fermented foods (*Bifidobacterium lactis, Lactobacillus acidophilus, Streptococcus thermophilus,* and more) that potentially provide a health benefit.

Interestingly, the species of bacteria typically used as probiotics are not "at home" in the gut. Scientists Justin Sonnenburg and Erica Sonnenburg, in their recent book *The Good Gut*, call probiotics "the transients" because they pass through the gut without taking up permanent residence. Nevertheless, growing mechanistic evidence suggests probiotics don't necessarily have to stick around to affect the resident microbes. In some cases they may positively affect immune system processes in the body. The question is whether they have any measurable effects on health.

Although results often conflict, researchers are amassing evidence for different benefits of probiotics—for reducing abdominal pain in irritable bowel syndrome, for curing travelers' diarrhea, for preventing antibiotic-associated diarrhea, and much more. Not all studies are considered high quality. In some cases, there is no placebo group to compare with the group that takes the probiotic, and in other cases the treatment groups are too small to draw conclusions from. Studies on the same probiotic strains sometimes come up with completely different results, making it difficult to see strong patterns and zero in on the most effective strain(s) and dose for each condition. Nevertheless, there is an overall pattern of benefit for probiotics, and the task facing scientists is to figure out how personalized probiotic treatments can address specific health conditions.

Prebiotics

Prebiotics—food for microbes—are a purified form of dietary fiber your body cannot absorb. Their claim to fame is helping the growth and activities of certain bacterial species that promote health. Prebiotics may induce longer-lasting positive change in the gut microbiome than probiotics.

Some of the common prebiotics are awkwardly named: oligofructose and inulin, for instance, as well as fructo-oligosaccharides and galacto-oligosaccharides. These are compounds found in (or derived from) foods such as asparagus, banana, and artichoke. Over time, researchers have recognized more and more substances that have prebiotic potential, and some researchers have constant debates over what falls into the prebiotic category.

Synbiotics

Synbiotics are combinations of probiotics and prebiotics delivered in one tidy package in food or supplement form. By delivering both the live microorganisms and the food they need to grow, synbiotics are said to have effects greater than the sum of their parts. The research on synbiotics is very thin, so it will be many years before we know how effective they are compared to probiotics or prebiotics alone.

PROBIOTIC SUPPLEMENTS: ARE THEY WORTH IT?

Say you ask your doctor about some symptoms and your doctor says, "Yes, go to the pharmacy and get some medicine. That should help you." Then she immediately walks out of the room, ending your consultation. You'd probably want to ask, "Wait, what kind of medicine? Shouldn't I pick something that's been tested for my condition?"

Like the word *medicine*, the word *probiotic* is very general. When deciding whether or not to take a probiotic supplement, it is essential to know what you are trying to treat and which strains are able to treat it. For example, there is a growing consensus that acute diarrhea and necrotizing enterocolitis in premature babies can be treated effectively with certain probiotic strains.[14] You can find the most up-to-date research and consumer infographics on the website of the International Scientific Association for Probiotics and Prebiotics, isappscience.org. They also release annual clinical guides to probiotic supplements that are available in Canada (probioticchart.ca) and in the United States (usprobioticguide.com).

It becomes more complicated if you want to take probiotics preventively. The science fails to back most claims that probiotics prevent illness—with the possible exception of upper respiratory tract infections and diarrhea that accompanies antibiotics. Probiotics do affect the immune system in various ways, but time will tell whether this means they protect you from a range of infections and conditions.

The biggest advantage of taking live bacteria in supplement form is that you know which strains you are delivering to your intestines in what (large) quantity. Because probiotic supplements can be pricey and the quality purportedly varies dramatically from brand to brand, it is best to do your research and check expiration dates. A good quality probiotic is refrigerated to preserve the life of the microorganisms, so they are alive when you consume them.

Microbiome Dietary Guidelines

The power of diet to affect the microbiome is emphasized by a number of recently published diet and lifestyle books that focus on improving the gut microbial community. These books all try to provide practical advice on how to change your lifestyle based on growing knowledge about the gut microbiome. *The Good Gut* by Justin Sonnenburg and Erica Sonnenburg thoroughly covers the science in this area. Robynne Chutkan's *The Microbiome Solution* skims through studies and offers general guidelines on diet. Other books stick less to the science and more to their clinical experience and intuition to develop very specific phases and diet plans, such as Gerard Mullin's *Gut Balance Revolution* and Raphael Kellman's *The Microbiome Diet*.

Here's the truth that you won't find in most microbiome diet books: as of 2016, scientists don't have all the answers. A food may be associated with the growth of certain bacteria, and that bacteria can be associated with a certain state of health, but it's not a fixed and predictable relationship.

With every week that goes by, however, scientists learn more about how to tailor what we eat to support the health of both our gut microbiomes and our bodies. And everyone has to eat, so it makes sense to eat the things known to effect positive change in the gut microbiome.

There are five main dietary guidelines, drawn from the science, for cultivating a diverse collection of bacterial species and positively affecting your gut microbiome:

1. **Choose carbohydrates wisely:** Starchy carbohydrates starve your microbes—ample evidence shows that increasing complex carbohydrates (fiber) helps them thrive.

2. **Eat meat in limited quantities:** Gut microbes assist in metabolizing meat components into potentially harmful substances.

3. **Limit saturated fat intake:** The microbes that proliferate with a high intake of saturated fat are associated with inflammatory processes and negative health outcomes.

4. **Consume beneficial bacteria:** Beneficial bacteria can come in food or supplement form.

5. **Avoid processed foods:** Many processed foods contain ingredients that, when studied in isolation, have detrimental effects on the guts of mice and humans. These include emulsifiers (polysorbate 80) and some artificial sweeteners (saccharin).

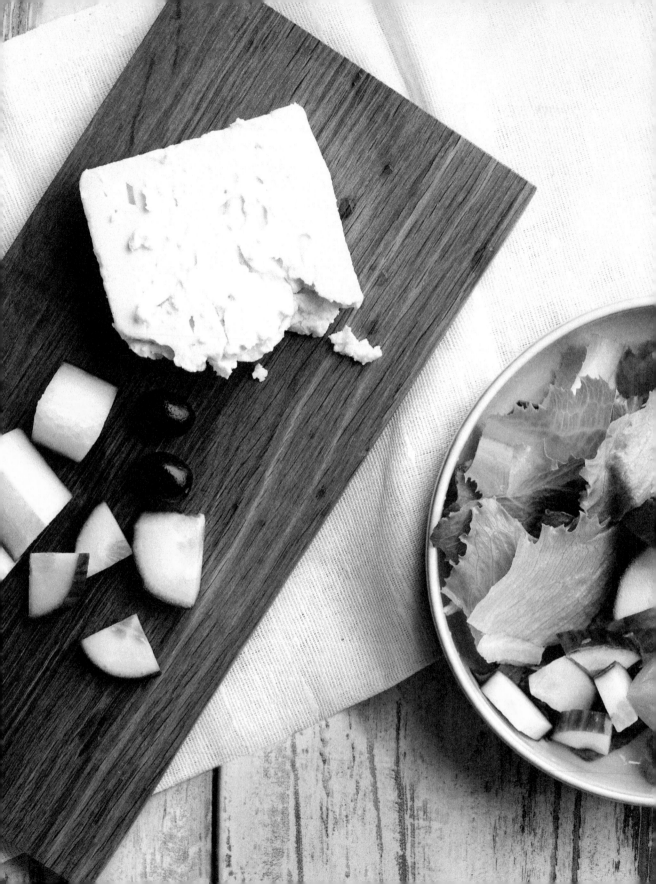

AN OVERVIEW
OF THE MICROBIOME
DIET PLAN

Now that you understand the vital importance of your gut microbiome to your health, it's time to take action. This chapter translates the general, science-based guidelines from chapter 1 into a plan you can use today. It covers the phases of the Microbiome Diet plan, foods that will become your best allies in maintaining microbial diversity, and lifestyle changes that will keep your gut microbes working for you rather than against you.

TWO PHASES: REPAIR AND REVITALIZE

The foods you eat are important in shaping your gut microbiome composition and health. The end goal of the Microbiome Diet plan is to help you nourish a diverse collection of gut microbes through a balanced diet that lets you take pleasure in your food. The foods listed in the "avoid" section will be eliminated because of the havoc they wreak on the gut, but this doesn't mean you have to suffer. This book provides an array of delicious options to suit both phases of the Microbiome Diet plan.

The scientific research on how diet affects health through the gut microbiome focuses on two different populations: people who have certain diseases or conditions, and people who are healthy. To parallel these categories, the Microbiome Diet action plan is divided into two phases.

Phase 1: Repair: The first phase is designed for people seeking relief from particular gut symptoms, such as frequent gas, bloating, abdominal pain, and diarrhea. The goal is to "change the filter" by altering your gut microbiome and giving it the best chance of supporting your health. You will probably need to accompany this diet phase with other lifestyle changes, which are detailed at the end of the chapter.

Phase 2: Revitalize: If you don't have any particular gut symptoms you are trying to address, you should jump right into Phase 2 of the Microbiome Diet plan. The second phase is for those who are generally healthy and want to keep their gut microbiome diverse to lay the groundwork for a reasonable weight and further good health. Although this part of the diet plan is presented as a "phase" to make it distinct from the diet designed to address digestive symptoms, Phase 2 is ideally a long-term proposition—it is a new way of eating to support your health for years to come.

The Microbiome Diet is the result of careful review of the literature on the foods that change the microbiome in ways that are beneficial to health. It is a practical take on the best available science. But it wouldn't be science if it were set in stone. In the fast-moving field of gut microbiome research, important new studies emerge every week. The finer details may change as scientists learn more from ongoing experiments. To stay up-to-date, you can check for periodic updates on the Intestinal Gardener blog (intestinalgardener.blogspot.ca).

One other note: Just as you personalize your diet every day—avoiding things you dislike and that sap your energy—you will likely personalize the Microbiome Diet plan. If you are allergic to any of the suggested foods in the recipes, of course, substitute another item. Many of the recipes include suggestions on adapting them to your own needs and preferences. In the future, doctors may have access to advanced methods for personalizing your diet according to what your gut microbiome requires. Researchers from Israel recently reported a large-scale study in which they gathered a patient's data, including his gut microbiome composition, and developed a mathematical model that helped predict which foods would spike the patient's blood sugar.[15] They used this information to recommend a personalized diet that kept blood sugar stable and was conducive to weight loss. The foods that kept blood sugar stable were sometimes surprising—for example, one patient was allowed to have ice cream and chocolate but had to give up grapes and salmon. More research is needed to figure out how to explain this phenomenon. Until this precise personalization is widely available, a local health professional may be able to help you meet your specific needs with a diet that is gut-microbe friendly.

PHASE 1: REPAIR

More physicians are realizing the power of diet to complement existing treatments for disease. Dr. Drew Ramsey, author of *The Happiness Diet*, for example, reports that in his psychiatry practice he regularly gives nutritional suggestions in addition to treatments, such as medication and talk therapy. Ramsey gives each patient a "brain food prescription" that lists foods, such as mussels or kale, specifically chosen to meet the patient's nutritional needs.

Building on the idea that the right foods can make a difference, the first phase of the Microbiome Diet plan is designed to suit someone trying to reduce distressing digestive symptoms, such as abdominal pain, gas, and bloating. It is based on two diets that have been tested in the scientific literature—the low-FODMAP diet and the IBD-AID:

- FODMAP is an acronym for a group of carbohydrates: "fermentable oligosaccharides, disaccharides, monosaccharides, and polyols." The **low-FODMAP diet**, developed by researchers at Monash University in Australia, minimizes consumption of these kinds of poorly absorbed carbohydrates.

Evidence from well-designed scientific studies shows that the low-FODMAP diet reduces symptoms of irritable bowel syndrome—abdominal pain, gas, and bloating—and also tiredness.[16] Preliminary research is also exploring this diet for those with inflammatory bowel disease (IBD). Evidence suggests that, for this group, it may lead to improvements in stool frequency and consistency, as well as reducing abdominal pain, gas, and bloating.[17] A 2014 study confirmed that the low-FODMAP diet does significantly change your gut microbiome, and this may be the way it achieves the reduction of symptoms.[18]

- Researchers at the University of Massachusetts Medical School used the specific carbohydrate diet as the basis for developing the **IBD-AID** (inflammatory bowel disease anti-inflammatory diet). The theoretical basis of this diet is to increase anti-inflammatory gut bacteria and decrease pro-inflammatory gut bacteria, restoring balance to the gut environment. This diet has not been well tested, but it shows promise in reducing IBD symptoms, including the frequency of bowel movements, and in allowing patients to discontinue some of the IBD medications they were previously taking.[19]

Phase 1 builds on these two medically useful diets. It uses the low-FODMAP diet as a base and adds moderate amounts of the fermented foods recommended in the IBD-AID. A few restrictions follow from recent research on maintaining general good health. Most studies require subjects to adhere to a low-FODMAP diet for three to six weeks. This book provides support for four weeks of the Phase 1 diet plan; you can extend this phase if needed.

Symptoms are the starting point of this phase. Both the low-FODMAP diet and the IBD-AID serve the best chance of reducing gastrointestinal symptoms that trouble patients the most, and they probably do this work, in part, by changing the gut microbiome. It's important to note that this phase of the diet may help symptoms, but it does not purport to cure these conditions or replace other therapies.

If you are relatively healthy and do not suffer from any gastrointestinal symptoms, such as the ones just detailed, you probably want to skip Phase 1 and move directly into Phase 2.

Foods to Avoid

Certain substances are avoided in both phases of the Microbiome Diet plan because they are, according to the best evidence available, detrimental to your health. You have probably heard some of these culprits mentioned elsewhere: processed meats, juices and sodas, and things that contain trans fats or refined sugars. Emulsifiers and artificial sweeteners are also avoided in this phase because new research shows they have specific negative effects on the gut microbiome. These items are found in many processed and packaged foods, from granola bars to ketchup, so this essentially means you have to commit to making your own foods for the duration of this diet plan. Fortunately, the recipes in the following chapters give you many delicious options.

Several other foods deserve mention. Potatoes are eliminated from Phase 1, since increased potato consumption is linked with low microbial gene richness and high systemic inflammation. Corn is also thought to increase inflammation through the gut microbiome, according to the University of Massachusetts researchers that developed the IBD-AID. Corn, flaxseed, soybean, and sunflower oils are avoided because new research shows they may contribute to inflammation.

Foods to Limit

Phase 1 requires eating beef, pork, and lamb in moderation. The jury is still out on exactly how red meat affects the gut microbiome, whether positively, neutrally, or negatively, but one line of research led by Stanley Hazen at Cleveland Clinic shows it may lead to bacteria producing a by-product called trimethylamine N-oxide (TMAO), which changes cholesterol metabolism and is implicated in cardiovascular disease. In this phase, all saturated fats are generally limited; however, small amounts of saturated fats (coconut oil, for example) are used in some recipes that require cooking at a higher heat.

Foods to Enjoy

Most low-FODMAP foods are enjoyed in Phase 1 of the Microbiome Diet plan. Allowed foods include certain dairy products, protein from chicken, eggs, fish, and shellfish, and many kinds of nuts, as well as oats and several other grains. Low-FODMAP fruits and vegetables are a big component of this phase. Maple syrup is suitable as a low-FODMAP sweetener. The table on pages 44–45 provides a detailed list of foods to avoid, limit, and enjoy during Phase 1. Not every possible food is on this list, however; in this phase, it can be helpful to download the Monash University Low FODMAP Diet smartphone app, which is updated regularly based on the latest food analysis. Through the app, you can conveniently check the FODMAP content of many foods not listed in the table. Remember, though, there are a few low-FODMAP foods still restricted in Phase 1 of the Microbiome Diet plan, and that in this phase, fermented foods such as yogurt are allowed if you tolerate them well.

Studies associate turmeric with health benefits through the microbiome, so this is an excellent spice to enjoy in this first diet phase. Low-FODMAP varieties of tea (black, green, and peppermint) are allowed, as well as moderate amounts of coffee if you are accustomed to drinking it.

When it comes to dietary fats, new research shows the *kind* of fat matters more for health than the *amount* of fat. So don't worry about counting grams of fat for your microbiome's sake. In this phase, focus primarily on consuming the mono-unsaturated fats in extra virgin olive oil and avocado, which are specifically associated with decreased markers of inflammation.

What to Expect During Phase 1

The Phase 1 restrictions may seem daunting at first. Good-bye coffee shop muffin. Good-bye quick slice of pizza at lunchtime. But don't be discouraged. If you keep careful track of your symptoms, you may be encouraged by the positive changes you see. People with IBS-like symptoms often say they experience dramatic changes within a week. And even if you don't see changes that quickly, you can bet you are changing your microbial community, helping shape it with every meal.

Tips for Success

Here's how to ensure that Phase 1 of the Microbiome Diet plan is a success:

Don't let yourself feel hungry. Fill up on reasonable portions of the foods allowed in this phase.

Invest time in planning your next meal or snack. That way, you're not tempted to eat foods on the "avoid" list. The lists in this book make it easy for you to plan so you have what you need on hand.

Put restricted foods out of sight, out of mind. Comb through your cupboards and remove things you won't be consuming in this phase of the diet.

Keep it simple. Life can be busy. If you don't have time to prepare the suggested meal one day, just find something on the "enjoy" list that's quick and easy; for example, an avocado and a tomato can serve as lunch in a pinch.

Tell others what you're doing. You'll be more likely to adhere to the plan if you have others cheering you on.

Practice self-compassion. Dwell on the positive changes you are making and thank yourself for your beautiful efforts to improve your health.

PHASE 2: REVITALIZE

Experiments suggest that your gut microbiome plays a role in determining your weight. Important pioneering work from Jeffrey Gordon's lab transplanted germ-free mice (i.e., those without bacterial populations in their digestive tracts) with the gut microbes of human twin pairs: one lean and one obese. Mice that received the gut microbes from the obese twin gained more weight. If mice that received the obese twin's microbes were then exposed to the lean twin's microbes, they didn't gain weight—as long as they were consuming a healthy diet.

So how do gut microbes determine human weight? You can bet scientists are staying late in their labs to figure this out. No one has yet been able simply to increase a "beneficial" strain of bacteria found in lean people and watch the pounds melt off. Practically speaking, the evidence suggests it's better to forget about miracle bacteria and focus on achieving diversity in your gut microbiome.

The name of the game in Phase 2 of the Microbiome Diet plan is *diversity*. As we learned in chapter 1, a diverse gut microbiome leads to better health—it's associated with lower weight and a lower risk of certain diseases.

Phase 2 of the Microbiome Diet plan is based on an overall dietary pattern associated with good health (a Mediterranean-style diet), plus specific foods that foster growth of a diverse collection of bacteria. There is no longer a restriction of FODMAPS; fruit, legumes, and vegetables are generally increased, as they modulate the microbiota and increase markers of good health. Fermented foods, such as yogurt, are important elements of this second diet phase. Increased consumption of both fiber and yogurt are associated with a lower body weight in large-scale population studies, and, furthermore, these food items appear to contribute to a thriving community of gut microbes.

"Eat more fiber" seems like the oldest health advice in the book. But it turns out fiber is your main ally in achieving microbial diversity. An intriguing study from Hehemann and colleagues showed that Japanese people who often ate seaweed had populations of special seaweed-digesting microbes in their guts.[20] It could be that each different fiber-rich food makes a meal for a different kind of microbe. So, if you eat fiber from a variety of sources, you'll help many kinds of microbes thrive.

Even though it's not such a radical idea that dietary fiber is associated with weight loss and good health, it is radical to think that fiber may do its good work by changing the microbiome. All along, scientists haven't really understood how fiber worked to benefit the body, but it's now clear that microbes have a role to play in fiber's health-giving effects.

Short-chain fatty acids (SCFAs) are the little magical molecules that may be responsible for the beneficial effects of fiber. It works like this: When you eat nondigestible carbohydrates (fiber), they reach the colon intact. Your resident bacteria feast on them (by producing enzymes that chop up the fiber into smaller components) and produce SCFAs as waste products. Some of these SCFAs provide energy for the cells of the intestine and help keep the inner layer of the colon healthy, and others travel through the blood to different organs, where they serve as messengers or provide materials for important bodily processes.

Phase 2 of the Microbiome Diet plan is designed for relatively healthy people who want to eat in a way that is good for their microbes. If you are transitioning from Phase 1 (where certain types of fiber are restricted) to Phase 2 (where fiber intake is increased), you may want to work up to Phase 2 gradually. (See page 43 for suggestions.)

While the Phase 2 meal plan in this book provides support for two weeks of the Phase 2 diet, it need not be a phase with a definite end. Phase 2 is designed to be a lifestyle change sustainable for the long term. Once you get to the end of the recipes, apply your creativity to the guidelines in this book to feed your microbes for years to come.

Foods to Avoid

The list of foods to avoid is shorter in Phase 2 than in Phase 1. As before, processed meats, juices and sodas, trans fats, refined sugars, emulsifiers, and artificial sweeteners are on the "avoid" list. In addition, corn, soybean, and sunflower oils are still avoided because, even in healthy people, they are associated with increased markers of inflammation.

Foods to Limit

As in Phase 1, Phase 2 involves limited amounts of red meat. Refined wheat flour also falls into the category of foods to limit; it gets special attention here because you find it everywhere, from pizza crusts to sandwich bread, yet it is low in fiber, and therefore, poor food for your gut microbes. You can still enjoy a white hamburger bun from time to time, but it is best to make a habit of avoiding foods made from white flour.

Foods to Enjoy

The main idea in this phase of the diet is to increase consumption of dietary fiber from a variety of sources. You no longer need be constrained by FODMAPs, so you can eat a wider range of grains, fruits, and vegetables. Indeed, some foods avoided when following a low-FODMAP diet now become your best friends—particularly those with inulin and FOS, including bananas, leeks, asparagus, garlic, onions, and Jerusalem artichokes.

The other key in Phase 2 is to increase consumption of fermented foods, both dairy and vegetables. Since buying a lot of these artisan foods in the stores can be pricey, see chapter 11 for tips on how to make your own fermented foods inexpensively at home.

Raw (unpasteurized) honey is added to the list of allowable sweeteners. Red wine is now allowed in moderate amounts, and dark chocolate is highly recommended. Flaxseed oil is added to the list of allowable oils.

For a more detailed list of foods to avoid, limit, and enjoy during Phase 2, consult the following table.

What to Expect During Phase 2

If you've skipped Phase 1, you can jump right into Phase 2. Note, however, that switching from Phase 1 to Phase 2 of the Microbiome Diet plan means a huge increase in dietary fiber intake, which could lead to undesirable gastrointestinal symptoms. It's best to transition slowly, adding new foods one at a time. See page 43 for information on reintroducing foods gradually, or ask a local health professional for support.

Tips for Success

Here's how to make sure Phase 2 of the Microbiome Diet plan is smooth sailing:

Above all, think "fiber." When you're planning meals or looking for a snack, choose the option that offers the most fiber for your microbes. Better yet, eat different fiber-rich foods in one sitting (for example, almonds and a banana).

Prepare foods in quantity. You are more likely to reach for vegetables if they are already peeled and cut up in the refrigerator, so prepare extras of microbiome-friendly foods when you have a little more time.

When eating out, go simple. Everyone eats out from time to time; when you do, don't feel completely constrained by the menu. Politely request modifications that benefit your microbes and help you know exactly what you're eating. Often this means deconstructing your dinner; for example, you can ask for oil and vinegar on the side, rather than the standard salad dressing.

What Is "One Serving?"

Use the following comparisons as your guide when estimating a serving size of various foods.

- **2 to 3 ounces of meat, poultry, or fish** is about the size of a standard deck of cards
- **½ cup cooked grains or pasta** fits inside a cupcake wrapper
- **½ cup cut or whole fruit** is about the size of a tennis ball
- **½ cup cooked or raw hard vegetables** is about the size of a tennis ball
- **1 cup leafy greens** is about the size of a large adult's fist
- **1 ounce cheese** is about equal to 2 stacked dominos

Reintroducing Foods

After weeks on Phase 1, it's time to reintroduce foods into your diet. This means adding foods, one by one, in a controlled manner and tracking symptoms that occur. For those with gastrointestinal disorders, "trigger" foods are those regularly linked with unwanted symptoms. Reintroducing foods slowly can help you determine if you have trigger foods.

Phases 1 and 2 are very different. Phase 1 restricts fiber; Phase 2 is heavy on fiber. If you follow Phase 1 and suddenly switch to Phase 2, you might end up with undesirable symptoms. A slow phasing in of fiber and other foods may help you avoid gastrointestinal discomfort.

To begin reintroducing foods after Phase 1, follow these steps:

1. **Identify your "baseline" symptoms.** You can do this by writing down the symptoms you experience in Phase 1. Use the worksheet on page 49 to help you.

2. **Pick one food to challenge.** Choose a food you eliminated in Phase 1 (for example, one with slightly higher FODMAP content).

3. **Try a small amount of that food (a half portion).** Note the quantity, date, and any symptoms that occur within the next 24 hours (using the chart on page 49). If you experience new symptoms, that food may be a trigger. Restrict this kind of food again, noting whether the symptoms go away.

4. **If you don't experience symptoms within 24 hours of the new food, try a similar food or the same food in larger quantity.** If you remain symptom free, write "OK" in the analysis column.

PHASE ❶
MICROBIOME DIET FOODS TO ENJOY, LIMIT, AND AVOID

DAIRY PRODUCTS (full-fat for maximum benefit, unless specified otherwise in recipes)

AVOID

Buttermilk
Condensed milk
Custard
Milk (cow's and goat's)

Soft cheeses
  (cottage, ricotta)
Sour cream

ENJOY

Butter
Cream cheese
Half-and-half (18 percent)
Hard "artisan" cheeses
  (Cheddar, Colby, Parmesan,
  Swiss)

Lactose-free dairy products
Low-FODMAP soft cheeses
  (Brie, feta, mozzarella)
Whipping (35 percent) cream
Yogurt, plain (not fat-free)

FRUITS

AVOID

Apple
Apricot
Blackberry
Date
Dried fruit
Fig

Guava
Mango
Nectarine
Papaya
Peach
Pear

Persimmon
Plum
Prune
Watermelon

ENJOY

Banana
Blueberry
Cantaloupe
Cranberry
Grape
Honeydew

Kiwi
Lemon
Lime
Orange
  (mandarin, navel)
Passion fruit

Pineapple
Raspberry
Rhubarb
Strawberry

GRAINS

AVOID

Barley
Bulgur

Rye
Wheat

ENJOY

Gluten-free grains (buckwheat,
  oats, quinoa, tapioca)
Rice
Spelt

MEATS AND EGGS

AVOID

Processed meats
  (bacon, ham, lunch meats,
  pepperoni, salami)

LIMIT (one or fewer servings per day)

Red meats (beef, pork, lamb)

ENJOY

Chicken
Eggs

Fish
Shellfish

PHASE ❶
MICROBIOME DIET FOODS TO ENJOY, LIMIT, AND AVOID

LEGUMES, NUTS, AND SEEDS

AVOID

Beans (black, kidney)
Cashew
Flaxseed
Lentils
Pistachio
Soy (soy beans, soy milk)

ENJOY

Milk alternatives
    (almond, coconut, rice)
Nuts, unsalted
    (almonds, macadamia nuts,
    peanuts, pecans, pine nuts,
    walnuts)
Pumpkin seeds
Tempeh
Tofu

VEGETABLES

AVOID

Artichoke
Beet
Broccoli
Cauliflower
Celery
Corn
Garlic
Leek
Mushroom
Onion
Potato
Sugar snap peas
Sweet potato

ENJOY

Avocado
Bamboo shoots
Bell pepper
Bok choy
Brussels sprouts
Cabbage
Carrot
Cucumber
Eggplant
Green beans
Kale
Lettuce
Low-FODMAP
    fermented
    vegetables
    (sauerkraut)
Parsnip
Pumpkin
Radish
Rutabaga
Seaweed (nori)
Spinach
Sprouts
    (alfalfa, bean)
Squash
Tomato
Turnip
Water chestnut
Zucchini

SPICES, SWEETENERS, CONDIMENTS, AND OTHER

AVOID

Artificial sweeteners (acesulfame
    potassium, aspartame,
    saccharin, sucralose)
Emulsifiers
    (carboxymethylcellulose,
    polysorbate-80)
Juice
Oils with polyunsaturated fats
    (corn, flaxseed, soybean,
    sunflower)
Soda
Sugar (agave, high-fructose
    corn syrup, table sugar)
Trans fats (commercial pastry,
    partially hydrogenated
    vegetable oil, shortening)

LIMIT (one or fewer servings per day)

Coffee

ENJOY

Cocoa powder
Maple syrup
Nutritional
    yeast
Olive oil
Sesame oil
Soy sauce
Turmeric

PHASE ❷
MICROBIOME DIET FOODS TO ENJOY, LIMIT, AND AVOID

DAIRY PRODUCTS (full-fat for maximum benefit, unless specified otherwise in recipes)

ENJOY

Butter
Buttermilk
Cream cheese
Half-and-half (18 percent)
Hard "artisan" cheeses
  (Cheddar, Colby, Parmesan,
  Swiss)
Lactose-free dairy products

Low-FODMAP soft cheeses
  (Brie, feta, mozzarella)
Milk (cow's and goat's)
Soft cheeses
  (cottage, ricotta)
Sour cream
Whipping (35 percent) cream
Yogurt, plain (not fat-free)

FRUITS

ENJOY

Apple
Apricot
Banana
Blackberry
Blueberry
Cantaloupe
Cranberry
Date
Dried fruit
Fig
Grape

Guava
Honeydew
Kiwi
Lemon
Lime
Mango
Nectarine
Orange
  (mandarin, navel)
Peach
Pear

Papaya
Passion fruit
Persimmon
Pineapple
Plum
Prune
Raspberry
Rhubarb
Strawberry
Watermelon

GRAINS

AVOID

Refined wheat

ENJOY

Barley
Bulgur
Gluten-free grains (buckwheat,
  oats, quinoa, tapioca)
Rice
Rye
Spelt
Wheat (whole grain)

MEATS AND EGGS

AVOID

Processed meats (bacon, ham,
  lunch meats, pepperoni, salami)

LIMIT (one or fewer servings per day)

Red meats (beef, pork, lamb)

ENJOY

Chicken   Fish
Eggs   Shellfish

PHASE ❷
MICROBIOME DIET FOODS TO ENJOY, LIMIT, AND AVOID

LEGUMES, NUTS, AND SEEDS

ENJOY

Milk alternatives (almond, coconut, rice, soy)
Beans
Cashews
Flaxseed
Lentils

Nuts, unsalted (almonds, macadamia nuts, peanuts, pecans, pine nuts, walnuts)
Pistachios
Pumpkin seeds
Soy (soy beans, soy milk)
Tempeh
Tofu

VEGETABLES

ENJOY

Artichoke
Avocado
Bamboo shoots
Beet
Bell pepper
Bok choy
Broccoli
Brussels sprouts
Cabbage
Carrot
Cauliflower
Celery
Corn
Cucumber

Eggplant
Garlic
Green beans
Kale
Leek
Lettuce
Low-FODMAP fermented vegetables (sauerkraut)
Mushroom
Onion
Parsnip
Potato

Pumpkin
Radish
Rutabaga
Seaweed (nori)
Spinach
Sprouts (alfalfa, bean)
Squash
Sugar snap peas
Sweet potato
Tomato
Turnip
Water chestnut
Zucchini

SPICES, SWEETENERS, CONDIMENTS, AND OTHER

AVOID

Artificial sweeteners (acesulfame potassium, aspartame, saccharin, sucralose)
Emulsifiers (carboxymethylcellulose, polysorbate 80)
Juice
Oils with polyunsaturated fats (corn, soybean, sunflower)
Soda
Sugar (agave, high-fructose corn syrup, table sugar)
Trans fats (commercial pastry, partially hydrogenated vegetable oil, shortening)

LIMIT (up to 2 servings per day)

Coffee
Red wine

ENJOY

Chocolate (dark)
Cocoa powder
Honey (raw)
Maple syrup

Nutritional yeast
Olive oil
Sesame oil
Soy sauce
Turmeric

It's best to be patient during the food reintroduction process since you don't want to undo the hard work you put in during Phase 1. Some low-FODMAP guidelines suggest adding foods back into your diet over a period of several weeks—the process could take as long as six weeks.

For example, to reintroduce cow's milk after completing Phase 1, note your baseline symptoms on Monday. On Tuesday morning, add a few tablespoons of milk to your coffee or tea. If no new symptoms appear that day, consume half a cup of milk on your cereal on Wednesday. If still symptom-free on Thursday, drink a cup of milk on its own. This should give you a good idea of whether you can tolerate milk in Phase 2.

Remember, the data may not be neat and tidy. Symptoms could be linked to other health factors; don't worry if you have initially confusing results. Do your best to avoid foods that regularly trigger unwanted effects.

A GUT-FRIENDLY LIFESTYLE

A century ago, a North American woman would have lived very differently than one in the modern world. She might have woken up early and headed straight outside, where she would have exchanged microbes with goats and cows as she groomed and milked them. She might have brought the milk inside and consumed some of it unboiled, teeming with bacteria and enzymes. She probably washed her hands and face (but not necessarily the rest of her body) daily with homemade soap. And because she didn't have a refrigerator, she regularly consumed root cellar foods (like fermented sauerkraut) preserved with the help of live bacteria.

You probably don't want to adopt this lifestyle today; there are good reasons most people no longer live this way. But one thing is certain: the woman from a century ago had a much richer exposure to microbes in her daily life than most women do today.

Are people worse off, overall, with the reduced microbial exposures in a typical Western lifestyle? Microbiome researchers have gone deep into the Amazon and parts of Africa to examine the microbiomes of people living far from industrialized society—those whose lifestyles expose them to a much greater diversity of microbes. Without fail, the microbiomes of those groups are much more diverse than those living in the West. On one hand, this may mean that healthy people from nonindustrialized societies have superior microbiomes to healthy people

BASELINE SYMPTOMS

Date	Symptoms & Severity*

*Rate on a scale of 1 to 5, with 1 being mild and 5 being severe.

FOOD REINTRODUCTION CHART

Date	Food	Serving Size

Symptoms & Severity*	Analysis

*Rate on a scale of 1 to 5, with 1 being mild and 5 being severe.

from the West. On the other hand, it could just mean that the microbiomes of people living in the Amazon are adapted to their specific lifestyle, as the microbiomes of people living in the West are adapted to theirs. Regardless of how scientists answer this question, it seems that maintaining at least a minimum level of diversity in the gut microbiome is crucial: it is repeatedly linked to better health in scientific studies.

It's no surprise that our diets have changed dramatically within the past century. Unfortunately, we don't know the long-term impact many of these changes are having on our bodies and our health. The goal is to find clarity in our confusing world of processed and marketed foods, and to take advantage of the best technology for producing economical and convenient food, as long as it supports our best possible health. It's fascinating to think how, little by little, the study of our gut microbiota could bring us back around to what we really should eat—indeed, what we *evolved* to eat.

This book is a resource for helping you figure out, based only on the scientific studies as of early 2016, how to use diet as a tool for keeping your gut microbiome in good shape. It is important to understand that your microbial exposure is more than just diet, however. Here is a summary of lifestyle changes that will help support your health through your microbiome:

- Eat a diverse diet of whole foods (mainly plants)
- Consume beneficial bacteria (e.g., *Bifidobacterium lactis, Lactobacillus acidophilus,* and *Streptococcus thermophilus*) regularly
- Wash with soap and water instead of sanitizing
- Use antibiotics judiciously
- Control stress whenever possible
- Interact regularly with both animals and humans

The scientific progress is exciting, yet there's a lot still to be discovered and communicated. You don't just have to stand by and wait; you can do several things to help this field of science move forward:

Become a citizen scientist: Citizen scientists are regular people who make observations or gather scientific data from the world around them. Often, the data is an important component of a project led by a research scientist. See the Resources section for ideas on how you can participate in microbiome research from the comfort of your own home.

Watch your language: Be kind to bacteria when you speak about them. Most of us are used to thinking of bacteria as "bad" or "disgusting," but as you have seen in the last two chapters, nothing could be further from the truth. Bacteria need ambassadors. Language can shape our views of the world in subtle ways, so we would all benefit from using neutral or positive language about bacteria.

You have done it! You are now up-to-date on how to be a good steward of your microbial organ and keep it functioning well. You have taken control of your diet in a way that gives you the best chance of improving your health. There's only one thing left to do: raise a fork to the best available evidence and dig into these delicious Microbiome Diet recipes.

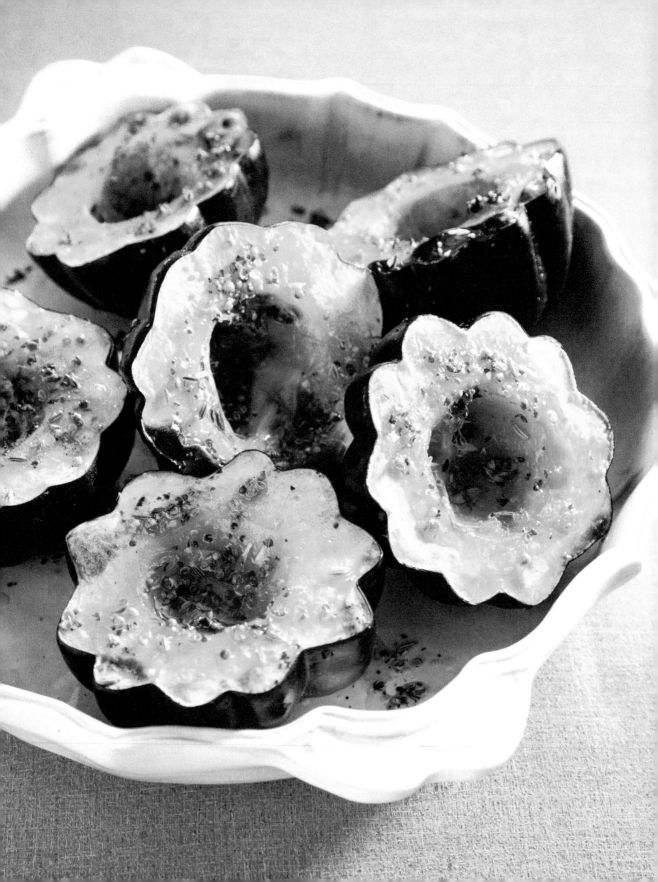

THE MICROBIOME DIET IN ACTION

You now know how important your gut colony is to overall health, so let's explore the delicious foods that will keep you and your microbiome feeling great. These simple, whole foods are packed with flavor and nutrients, and in Phase 1, they can provide healing relief. Remember, the Microbiome Diet is not about counting calories, but about eating healthful meals designed to optimize health. Whatever your kitchen experience, these tips and suggestions will help you easily transition to this diet.

Setting Yourself Up for Success

This transition to cooking and eating whole foods can be a bit overwhelming, especially if you are accustomed to convenience and processed foods. Cutting out these foods, along with sweetened beverages, is often the most difficult step of the journey, but it's one that will ultimately make you feel much better. Use the following tips to set yourself up to overcome all obstacles to changing your eating habits for good.

Shop once per week. One of the biggest keys to success for healthy eating is careful meal planning and shopping. The grocery lists and guides included in this chapter make it easy to follow for the first several weeks, and they get you in the habit of making a grocery list and using a meal plan. Follow along in Phase 1 and during the first two weeks of Phase 2, and you will begin to see how much time and money this way of preparing food saves you. There will be less wasted food, and you will be in and out of the store more quickly. By the time you are done with the first six weeks, you will be in the habit of making a grocery list that is made up of whole foods, and, by week seven, you will be ready to step out on your own and succeed in meal planning and shopping for your favorite recipes.

Cleanse your cupboards. It is a lot easier to stick with your diet when you don't have a bunch of processed foods, sweets, and other temptations staring you in the face every time you open your cupboards. Go through your pantry and get rid of any processed foods that contain ingredients not allowed on this diet. This will help jump-start your healthy lifestyle and remove unnecessary temptation. If you share cupboards with family or friends and don't want to toss everything that doesn't fit, designate a different area in the kitchen for these foods so you are not constantly looking at them when preparing meals.

Cook in bulk. Many recipes in this book yield four servings—perhaps a meal for one, with two or three additional servings for consuming at a later date. This saves you time in the kitchen and allows you a night off from cooking a few times a week—a definite treat, especially when adjusting to this new style of eating. If you cook for more people than just yourself, simply double the recipes as needed and save the remainder of the dish for the next serving.

Ferment foods yourself. Yes, you read that right! You really can make them yourself, and the bonus is you save quite a bit of money along the way. Fermentation is very easy, whether you have experience or not. All you need is a little instruction, a healthy dose of patience, a bit of attention to detail, and a few large glass jars. Follow our simple beginner-level recipes (pages 242–261) and be on your way to creating your very own fermented foods.

Hydrate. Your body is comprised of up to 60 percent water, and this water is instrumental in flushing waste, regulating body temperature, transporting nutrients, and lubricating joints. Replacing sugary sodas and juices with water is not only a great way to stay hydrated, but it is also a boon to weight-loss efforts— you will eliminate 140 calories per 12-ounce can of soda that you cut out. If you don't like plain water, add some lemon, orange, or lime slices; basil or cilantro leaves; or strawberry slices for added flavor. Herbal teas are also a great choice and can be a flavorful alternative to water or soda that will keep your taste buds satisfied.

Relax and enjoy. Did you know that chewing food enhances its digestion? The enzyme amylase, active in your saliva, is released as you chew and immediately begins to prepare carbohydrates to be digested. Slow down and savor your food, remembering to chew each bite thoroughly and enjoy it. As hard as it may be, sit down and enjoy your meal away from the computer, phone, work, or other distractions. Share your meals with friends and family and allow for a stress-free eating environment—you will enjoy the mealtime ritual all the more and reap the health benefits of slow, meaningful eating.

ESSENTIAL KITCHEN EQUIPMENT

Before you begin, you must first prepare your kitchen. The good news is that the Microbiome Diet is one of simplicity, and therefore, you do not need much to get started. In fact, you probably already have many, if not all, the items you need in your kitchen.

Pots and Pans

You will need a small or medium saucepan with a lid, as well as a 4-quart (or larger) stockpot to make many recipes in this book. You'll also need an 8-inch frying pan, a 12-by-18-inch baking sheet, and a large baking dish. Pots and pans made from nonreactive metal such as stainless steel are best, but ceramic, enameled, cast iron, glass, and other nonreactive metals work fine, too. Try to avoid nonstick-coated surfaces, as the lifespan of these items is limited, and the nonstick coating can easily become scratched, with possible negative health effects.

DIY HOME FERMENTATION

Foods have been fermented in home kitchens for hundreds of years, and they can be fermented easily in yours! Around the world, home cooks introduce myriad healthful bacteria cultivated in their very own kitchens into their guts, and you can, too. Home fermentation is a simple process you can start now with little equipment and just a few supplies.

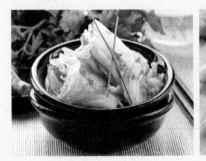
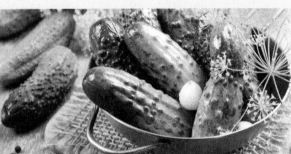

Asian countries are known for their bounty of fermented foods. From Korean kimchi to Japanese natto and miso, these delicious foods are part of everyday life in these traditional societies that practice food as medicine. Kefir, the fermented milk drink similar to yogurt, can be traced back over 2,000 years to Russia, while sauerkraut, popularly thought to be a German invention, was first made over 2,000 years ago in China using rice wine.

The initial purpose of fermentation was preservation; today, as its health benefits become more widely known, there are even more reasons to incorporate fermented foods into your diet.

Boutique fermented food companies are everywhere, but you can cut your fermented food bill in half by fermenting foods yourself. The process takes time, but this simple craft can easily be added to your daily regimen and subsequently improve your quality of life, making this diet accessible and affordable.

To ferment foods at home, you need just a few additional pieces of equipment and pantry staples.

CANNING AND PICKLING SALT

This is simply salt that does not contain iodide or additional additives to prevent caking. It is sold in 5-pound boxes and labeled "canning and pickling salt." While table salt will not harm the finished pickle, it will create an undesirable haze and sediment in the jar. If you cannot source canning and pickling salt, sea salt can be used. However, read the label to ensure there are no additives in the salt, as labeling laws on "sea salt" are unregulated. Do not use any colored sea salts, as these can create problems during fermentation.

NONREACTIVE FERMENTATION VESSELS

You will need one or two fermentation vessels for making fermented foods. These can be glass or other nonreactive containers, such as enameled stoneware. The vessels should have a wide mouth to allow for plenty of surface area contact with the air. Wide-mouth Mason jars are great for fermenting, and are probably the easiest and most inexpensive option. If you use Mason jars, an assortment of sizes is ideal, with wide-mouth quart and half-gallon jars being the most commonly used sizes for small-batch fermentation. If you enjoy fermenting foods in large batches, investing in a new crock made especially for this purpose is a great option, and plenty of inexpensive options are available, ranging from 1- to 6-gallon crocks.

STORAGE CONTAINERS

Once your foods finish fermenting, you will need something to store them in. If you fermented in Mason jars, transfer these to the refrigerator, capped with a nonreactive plastic lid. Look for plastic lids designed for Mason jars anywhere that Mason jars are sold. If you used another fermentation vessel, transfer the food to a Mason jar or another type of glass storage container.

BASIC TIPS FOR FERMENTATION

Keep it clean, but not too clean. Fermentation requires cleanliness to promote good bacteria and inhibit the bad. Always clean your workspace, utensils, and fermentation vessel with hot, soapy water, rinse thoroughly, and allow the items to air-dry before beginning any project. While clean hands are necessary, avoid the use of antibacterial soaps, which can inhibit bacterial growth. Do not clean counters, cutting boards, or utensils with antibacterial soaps either, as this can have the same effect—killing both the bad and good bacteria.

Maintain a watchful eye. While you don't need to check fermented foods several times a day, you also don't want to put them in a cupboard and forget about them. Store them in plain sight so you remember to peek in at them once a day during fermentation to correct any problems that may arise.

Keep it cool. Most fermented foods taste and perform best when fermented at a consistent temperature—between 65°F and 72°F. Fluctuations in temperature can speed up or slow down fermentation. During winter, a warm area of the kitchen is best to maintain this temperature, but in summer you may need to move your ferments to a cooler location, such as a basement, root cellar, or cool shed. Adjust fermentation locations seasonally to maintain a relatively constant temperature to get the most consistent results.

Small Appliances

For making smoothies, a high-powered blender is a great tool, especially when you plan to incorporate this diet into your life permanently. High-powered blenders grind fruits and vegetables into fine pieces, creating perfectly blended smoothies without graininess, which makes a big difference in quality. Fortunately, many types of these blenders are easily available, from the high-end (Vitamix) to the less expensive (NutriBullet, Nutri Ninja, and countless other varieties). If you don't want to make the investment now, a standard blender, or even an immersion blender, can be used to make smoothies until you are ready to invest more—just remember that you won't be able to achieve as smooth a texture.

For soups, a handheld immersion blender makes puréeing quick and easy, but a traditional blender works just as well.

Bowls and Measuring Cups

You will need mixing bowls for the preparation of many recipes in this book. Having a few of these bowls in different sizes is helpful and makes prep time simpler. You will need standard measuring cups and spoons. Glass measuring cups are great for measuring liquids by volume, and stainless steel or plastic measuring cups and spoons work well for dry goods.

Cooking Utensils and Other Tools

For mixing, cooking, and serving, you will need a couple of good spoons and spatulas. Choose wood, stainless steel, or other nonreactive metal spoons and spatulas when possible.

A small fine-mesh stainless steel strainer is also a helpful tool to have on hand, as are a box grater, vegetable peeler, and colander. A small steamer basket that fits into one of your pots is also necessary for some recipes.

Storage Containers

For some recipes, you will prepare a large amount of protein such as chicken on one day, and then use the leftover chicken over the course of two or three days. In these cases, you will need some airtight containers to store leftovers and food for later in the week. Glass is desirable, but food can also be stored in food-safe plastic containers. Mason jars also work great and are a cost-effective solution for storing soups, smoothies, and even salads. You will need up to 6 pint-size containers at one time when freezing chicken stock for meals later in the month, as well as a few more containers for storing leftovers.

PANTRY STAPLES

You don't need a bunch of fancy ingredients for the Microbiome Diet. However, a well-stocked pantry will go a long way to help prepare these meals easily. You don't need to get everything on the list, but these are some of the most commonly used dry pantry goods you will need to get started.

Nuts, Nut Butters, and Seeds

When stocking up on these items, remember some have a longer shelf life than others. In cases where the shelf life may be shorter, buy only what you need for that week's menu.

Almond butter: Organic almond butter is the best option, and there are numerous types available. Look for a natural variety without any added hydrogenated oils. Because almond butter becomes rancid more quickly than peanut butter, buy a small container.

Almonds: Select raw organic almonds when possible to avoid pesticide exposure. Buy whole almonds with their skin on to protect against rancidity for longer storage. If a recipe calls for toasted almonds, do this yourself at home.

Chia seeds: You can find these at many natural and health food stores. In some places, they are also sold in bulk bins. They should be refrigerated to preserve freshness.

Macadamia nuts: Raw macadamia nuts should be a white color when you buy them, as a yellowing indicates they are becoming rancid. For the best product, look for organic nuts packaged in a vacuum-sealed bag.

Natural peanut butter (smooth or chunky, as desired): Look for organic peanut butter that contains only peanuts and salt, or just peanuts. Avoid peanut butters with hydrogenated oils. You will have to stir a natural peanut butter before using to combine the separated oils from the peanuts.

Pistachios: Select plain, tan-colored raw organic pistachios over the red dyed variety. When mature, the nuts pop open the end of their shell, shortening their shelf life. If buying shelled pistachios, buy only what you need as they become rancid quickly.

Pumpkin seeds: Also called a pepita, the pumpkin seed is naturally a peculiar green color. They can be eaten both roasted and raw. (Choose organic whenever possible.)

Sunflower seeds: For salads, hulled raw organic sunflower seeds are often the quickest solution; though, like other seeds and nuts, their shelf life is decreased once they are removed from their shell. For this reason, it is recommended that you store hulled sunflower seeds in the refrigerator.

Walnuts: Whole walnuts in the shell have the most flavor (choose organic whenever possible), but having halved, quartered, and pieces of raw walnuts on hand makes adding them to meals simpler. If you don't want to buy more than one type, opt for the halves and crush them yourself as needed based on recipe directions.

Oils/Fats

Here is the list of the most commonly used healthy fats in this book's recipes.

Coconut oil: Unrefined coconut oil is available in many major grocery stores. It is great for baking and can be substituted for butter in most recipes. It does not need to be refrigerated.

Olive oil: This is the main oil used throughout this book. Choose pure extra virgin olive oil. There are many types of olive oil available. For cooking, a mildly flavored oil works well, while a salad can benefit from a more robustly flavored oil.

Sesame oil: This oil is used in many Asian dishes and is widely used throughout this book. Look for pure sesame oil; avoid any mixed with other oils.

Herbs and Spices

The following herbs and spices are the ones most commonly used throughout this book.

Asafetida	Cinnamon, ground	Dill, dried
Black peppercorns	Coriander, ground	Ginger, fresh and ground
Cardamom pods, green	Cumin, ground	Nutmeg, ground
Cayenne pepper	Curry powder	Oregano, dried

Pickling salt	Sea salt	Turmeric, fresh
Poppy seeds	Thyme, dried	and dried
Red pepper flakes		White peppercorns

Other Items

Apple cider vinegar: Look for organic apple cider vinegar that contains live cultures for the best flavor and benefit. Many types of apple cider vinegar are simply flavored white vinegar; read the label.

Baking powder

Baking soda

Balsamic vinegar: This sweet-sour vinegar is dark reddish-brown in color and is the ultimate in flavor. Traditional balsamic vinegar, made in Modena, Italy, is aged for at least 12 years; most widely available varieties are short-fermented but still complex in flavor.

Coconut, dried and unsweetened, shredded and flaked: Coconut is available both sweetened and unsweetened in many forms: finely shredded as well as in larger flakes. (Flaked coconut is great in granola, trail mix, and on cereals.) Choose unsweetened dried coconut for the recipes in this book to avoid unwanted sugar.

Coconut flour: This has a light coconut flavor and can be partially substituted for wheat-based flours in baked goods.

Dijon mustard: Look for a high-quality Dijon mustard free from preservatives, sugar, and, most important in Phase 1, powdered garlic or onions.

Maple syrup: Pure maple syrup is the primary natural sweetener called for in this diet, and you should keep a bottle on hand at all times to sweeten sauces, dressings, and desserts.

Nutritional yeast: Made from pasteurized yeast, nutritional yeast has a pleasant, nutty, cheese-like flavor. Look for it in health and natural food stores.

Red wine vinegar: This inexpensive vinegar is used predominantly in salad dressings. Look for one that does not contain a lot of preservatives.

Rice: Keep a selection of brown and white rice on hand for different dishes.

Rice vinegar: Made from white rice, this mild-tasting vinegar works well on salads and in dressings. Look for it in the Asian section of your grocery store.

Soy sauce: This is widely used as a flavoring agent throughout the recipes in this book. While typical soy sauce is fine in both Phase 1 and Phase 2 of the diet, if you have a gluten sensitivity, choose tamari soy sauce, as it is wheat free (check the label).

Whole-grain mustard: These mustards are thick and contain whole mustard seeds. They have a robust flavor and are great for flavoring soups, stews, and other liquid-based dishes.

Vanilla extract (pure): Pure vanilla is made from only two ingredients: vanilla beans and alcohol. Always choose pure vanilla extract to avoid unwanted chemical additives and sweeteners, such as corn syrup and sugar.

SHOPPING SUGGESTIONS

Staying on task and sticking with your diet can be difficult, especially in the beginning when this may be an entirely new way of eating for you. Many distractions can stand in your way, so the goal is to eliminate some of those distractions and give you the tools to succeed. Whether you are on Phase 1 or Phase 2, these simple steps can help you save money, make better food choices, and avoid temptation at the grocery store, leading to an all-around healthier you.

Shop the Perimeter

The perimeter of the grocery store is where many of the healthy items that you will be focusing on in this diet are situated. You will find produce, meats, and dairy products in refrigerated cases and shelves that line the exterior of the grocery store. You can skip over most of the interior aisles where the processed foods and junk foods are stocked. This will cut down on your shopping time and help you avoid the temptation to pick up any items you shouldn't be eating.

Go Prepared

Just as you don't go to a meeting or interview unprepared, you shouldn't go to the grocery store unprepared. Plan what you buy so you stay on task—and don't go hungry, lest low blood sugar persuade you to make rash decisions. Plan to shop after a meal, or bring a small portable snack such as a handful of nuts or a piece of fruit to stave off hunger.

Buy in Bulk

With most products, the larger the quantity you purchase, the better the price. Whether you are buying meat, spices, or olive oil, these savings add up and also help keep your refrigerator or freezer and pantry stocked. Get in the habit of buying a large package of chicken, splitting it into the portions needed for your recipes, and storing it to have it on hand when you need it. Seek out a store that sells dry items out of bulk bins, as these are often cheaper than the packaged varieties and allows you to buy even smaller quantities at a cost savings.

Read Labels

Since you will be preparing most of the foods you eat from scratch, this won't apply to 90 percent of your shopping trip. However, it does apply when purchasing fermented foods. It is highly recommended that you try your hand at fermentation, but chances are you will buy a few fermented foods from the grocery store. Look for natural, unpasteurized fermented foods that list "live cultures" on the label, and avoid products that are heat processed or pickled using vinegar.

THE RECIPES

The recipes in this book feature fresh, whole ingredients. While highly processed and convenience foods are avoided, some ingredients, such as grains and dairy products, are minimally processed before packaging. With recipes inspired from dishes around the world, you'll be able to put simple and delicious meals on the table in under an hour, with many dishes taking less than 20 minutes to prepare.

All recipes are labeled as either Phase 1 or Phase 2, depending on their respective ingredients. In some cases, substitution tips have been included so you can tailor the recipe to Phase 1 or Phase 2 (and vice versa), as needed. Follow these suggestions or choose substitutions from the food charts on pages 64–69. Adventurous home cooks can even assemble entire meals by simply using the food charts as a guide.

Recipes are labeled as applicable (Vegetarian, Vegan, Dairy-Free, Grain-Free, Gluten-Free, Nut-Free, Soy-Free, Kid-Friendly, Low-FODMAP) to help you easily identify whether a recipe is right for you. While many of the "big 8 allergens" (fish, tree nuts, peanuts, dairy, eggs, shellfish, soy, and wheat) are used throughout this book, you'll find many suggestions for substitutions so you can tailor dishes to suit your personal needs.

Following are 4 weeks of meal plans to get you solidly started on Phase 1.

	Breakfast	Lunch	Dinner	Snack
Day One	Quinoa, Buckwheat & Oat Granola (page 79) with Yogurt (page 258)	Greek Salad (page 111)	Salmon Patties (page 152), Sautéed Greens with Pine Nuts (page 123), and fermented vegetables	Popped Corn (page 203)
Day Two	Fruity Yogurt, Nut & Seed Parfait (page 78)	Kale & Walnut Salad (page 114) and fermented vegetables	Peanut-Ginger Chicken Soba Noodles (page 175)	Handful of walnuts and ½ cup of blueberries
Day Three	Parmesan-Basil Scrambled Eggs (page 90)	Creamy Tomato & Spinach Soup (page 104)	"Butter" Chicken (page 176) with rice; fermented vegetables	Hardboiled egg with sea salt and pepper
Day Four	Green Breakfast Smoothie (page 75)	Parmesan-Quinoa Patties & Spinach Salad (page 116)	Pesto Baked Chicken (page 179), Rutabaga Fries (page 129), and fermented vegetables	Handful of Super Nutty Trail Mix (page 199)
Day Five	Steel-Cut Oatmeal with Nuts & Fruit (page 83)	Curried Chicken Soup (page 108)	Quinoa & Roasted Vegetable Bowl (page 136) and Spiced Lassi (page 260)	Handful of walnuts and 1 kiwi
Day Six	Feta & Spinach Omelet (page 92)	Harvest Salad (page 112) and fermented vegetables	Curried Coconut Whitefish (page 160) with rice and Sautéed Greens with Pine Nuts (page 123)	Kale Chips (page 206)
Day Seven	Oatmeal Waffles (page 89)	Chicken Salad Wraps (page 172) and Hot & Spicy Pickles (page 251) or Dill Pickles (page 249)	Whole Roasted Mackerel (page 157), Turmeric-Spiced Quinoa Salad (page 139), and Sautéed Swiss Chard with Balsamic Vinegar (page 124)	2 slices Cheddar cheese and a handful of walnuts

	Breakfast	Lunch	Dinner	Snack
Day One	Coconut Teff Porridge (page 81)	Broccoli & Spinach Cheddar Soup (page 103) and Pickled Daikon (page 248), Hot & Spicy Pickles (page 251), or Dill Pickles (page 249)	Broiled Sole with Orange, White Wine & Dill (page 155) and Sautéed Greens with Pine Nuts (page 123)	Handful of gluten-free pretzels and a handful of blueberries
Day Two	Peanut Butter–Chocolate Breakfast Bars (page 80)	Salmon Salad Lettuce Wraps (page 149) and Pickled Daikon (page 248), Hot & Spicy Pickles (page 251), or Dill Pickles (page 249)	Chicken Kebabs (page 180) with rice and Greek Salad (page 111)	Radish slices topped with almond butter
Day Three	Savory Steel-Cut Oatmeal with Spinach (page 84)	Pumpkin Soup (page 101)	Oven-Baked Crispy Chicken Wings (page 184), Roasted Butternut Squash (page 125), and fermented vegetables	2 slices hard cheese and a handful of red or green grapes
Day Four	Blueberry-Coconut Quinoa Breakfast Bowl (page 85)	Cobb Salad (page 113) and fermented vegetables	Family Cabbage Casserole (page 193)	1 mandarin orange
Day Five	Almond-Banana Smoothie (page 77)	Tom Kha Gai (page 110)	Tuna & Quinoa Patties (page 154), Kale & Walnut Salad (page 114), and fermented vegetables	Handful of Maple-Cayenne Roasted Almonds (page 201)
Day Six	Quinoa, Buckwheat & Oat Granola (page 79) with Yogurt (page 258)	Leftover Family Cabbage Casserole	Green Curry Chicken (page 186) with rice; fermented vegetables	Deviled Eggs (page 208)
Day Seven	Banana Oat Pancakes (page 86)	Parmesan-Quinoa Patties & Spinach Salad (page 116)	Turkey Breast with Herbs (page 189) and Mashed Celeriac (page 130)	½ cup diced honeydew melon

	Breakfast	Lunch	Dinner	Snack
Day One	Creamy Millet Porridge (page 82)	Chicken Vegetable Soup (page 107)	Turmeric Curried Salmon (page 151) with rice, Kale & Walnut Salad (page 114), and fermented vegetables	½ cup pineapple and a handful of nuts
Day Two	Blueberry-Melon Smoothie (page 76)	Thai-Style Whitefish Salad (page 161) and fermented vegetables	Miso Chicken & Buckwheat Soba Stir-Fry (page 174) and Spiced Kabocha Squash (page 127)	Hardboiled egg with sea salt and pepper
Day Three	Eggs "Benekraut" (page 94)	Greek Salad (page 111) and leftover Spiced Kabocha Squash	Salmon with Miso Sauce (page 150) and Vegetable Fried Rice (page 145)	2 slices hard cheese and a handful of red or green grapes
Day Four	Kimchi Omelet (page 93)	Creamy Avocado Soup (page 102) and fermented vegetables	Chicken & Rice Casserole (page 182)	Yogurt (page 258) with mandarin orange slices
Day Five	Quinoa, Buckwheat & Oat Granola (page 79) with Yogurt (page 258)	Leftover Chicken & Rice Casserole	Turkey Meatballs (page 188), Mashed Celeriac (page 130), and a green salad	Handful of gluten-free pretzels and 1 banana
Day Six	Feta & Spinach Omelet (page 92)	Chicken Salad Wraps (page 172) and Pickled Daikon (page 248), Hot & Spicy Pickles (page 251), or Dill Pickles (page 249)	Quinoa & Roasted Vegetable Bowl (page 136)	½ cup diced honeydew melon and a handful of Curried Walnuts (page 200)
Day Seven	Buckwheat Pancakes with Blueberry Sauce (page 87)	Leftover Quinoa & Roasted Vegetable Bowl; fermented vegetables	Roasted Pork Loin (page 192) and Sautéed Greens with Pine Nuts (page 123)	Handful of nuts and a handful of red or green grapes

	Breakfast	Lunch	Dinner	Snack
Day One	Fruity Yogurt, Nut & Seed Parfait (page 78)	Tuna & Quinoa Patties (page 154) and fermented vegetables	Mediterranean Sorghum Bowl (page 140)	Yogurt (page 258) with blueberries
Day Two	Steel-Cut Oatmeal with Nuts & Fruit (page 83)	Leftover Mediterranean Sorghum Bowl and fermented vegetables	Bok Choy & Macadamia Stir Fry (page 143) with rice	Hardboiled egg with sea salt and pepper
Day Three	Kimchi Omelet (page 93)	Salmon Salad Lettuce Wraps (page 149)	Tofu & Quinoa Bowl with Snap Peas (page 135) and fermented vegetables	Kale Chips (page 206)
Day Four	Berrylicious Fruit Salad (page 118)	Kale & Walnut Salad (page 114) and fermented vegetables	Lemon Shrimp (page 165), Sautéed Greens with Pine Nuts (page 123), and rice	Nori-Seasoned Popped Corn (page 203)
Day Five	Quinoa, Buckwheat & Oat Granola (page 79) with Yogurt (page 258)	Greek Salad (page 111) and fermented vegetables	Mediterranean Baked Whitefish (page 159) and a green salad	½ cup cantaloupe and 2 slices hard cheese
Day Six	Buckwheat Crêpes with Southwestern Scramble (page 88)	Harvest Salad (page 112) and fermented vegetables	Sea Scallops with Gremolata (page 167) and Kale & Walnut Salad (page 114)	1 mandarin orange
Day Seven	Buckwheat Pancakes with Blueberry Sauce (page 87)	Turmeric-Spiced Quinoa Salad (page 139) and fermented vegetables	Chicken Kebabs (page 180) with rice and fermented vegetables	Zucchini Chips (page 207)

Now that you've graduated to Phase 2, enjoy these additional foods in your diet.

	Breakfast	Lunch	Dinner	Snack
Day One	Feta & Spinach Omelet (page 92) with asparagus and Parmesan cheese	Black Bean Soup (page 105)	Whitefish Cakes (page 156), Roasted Jerusalem Artichokes (page 132), and fermented vegetables	Apple slices with almond butter
Day Two	Creamy Millet Porridge (page 82) with apples	Greek Salad (page 111) with beets; fermented vegetables	Salmon Patties (page 152) with peas and a green salad	Dried Strawberries (page 197)
Day Three	Kimchi Omelet (page 93)	Vegetable Millet Bowl & Tahini Dressing (page 141) with chickpeas	Chicken Parmesan (page 181), steamed or sautéed greens, and fermented vegetables	Jerusalem Artichoke Chips (page 205)
Day Four	Steel-Cut Oatmeal with Nuts & Fruit (page 83)	Lentil-Carrot Soup (page 106)	Sea Scallops with Gremolata (page 167) with garlic and Cauliflower Rice (page 133)	Roasted Asparagus (page 131)
Day Five	Quinoa, Buckwheat & Oat Granola (page 79) with Kefir (page 255)	Harvest Salad (page 112) with apples, celery, and cranberries	Slow Cooker Beef Stew (page 191)	Yogurt (page 258) with blueberries and honey
Day Six	Buckwheat Crêpes with Southwestern Scramble (page 88)	Leftover Slow Cooker Beef Stew	Easy Fish Pie (page 163)	Roasted Chickpeas (page 202)
Day Seven	Buckwheat Pancakes with Blueberry Syrup (page 87)	Broccoli & Spinach Cheddar Soup (page 103)	Sticky Chicken Wings (page 185) with Cauliflower Rice (page 133)	Celery stalk with peanut butter

	Breakfast	Lunch	Dinner	Snack
Day One	Eggs "Benekraut" (page 94) with whole-wheat toast	Creamy Parsnip Soup (page 109)	Spicy Beef Curry (page 190) with Cauliflower Rice (page 133)	Curried Walnuts (page 200)
Day Two	Quinoa, Buckwheat & Oat Granola (page 79) with Kefir (page 255) and berries	Kale & Pear Salad (page 115) and fermented vegetables	Zucchini Rice Boats (page 138)	Deviled Eggs (page 208)
Day Three	Fruity Yogurt, Nut & Seed Parfait (page 78) with raspberries, blackberries, and blueberries	Leftover Zucchini Rice Boats (page 138) and fermented vegetables	Salmon Baked with Herbs (page 153) and Roasted Asparagus (page 131)	1 small plum and a handful of nuts
Day Four	Steel-Cut Oatmeal (page 83) with nuts & peaches	Curried Chicken Soup (page 108) with peas	Smoked Mackerel, Potato & Arugula Salad (page 158) and fermented vegetables	Handful of Super Nutty Trail Mix (page 199)
Day Five	Blueberry-Coconut Quinoa Breakfast Bowl (page 85) with peaches	Black Bean Burgers (page 144) and Sautéed Swiss Chard with Balsamic Vinegar (page 124)	Roasted Pork Loin (page 192) with garlic, Spiced Kabocha Squash (page 127), and Sautéed Greens with Pine Nuts (page 123) and golden raisins	Jerusalem Artichoke Chips (page 205)
Day Six	Banana Oat Pancakes (page 86) with Strawberry Shortcake Syrup (page 231)	Chicken Salad Wraps (page 172) with grapes and celery, Pickled Daikon (page 248), Hot & Spicy Pickles (page 251), or Dill Pickles (page 249)	Buckwheat Tabbouleh with Avocado & Chickpeas (page 142)	Dried Bananas (page 198)
Day Seven	Parmesan-Basil Scrambled Eggs (page 90) with garlic	Kale & Pear Salad (page 115) and fermented vegetables	Chicken Chili (page 178) with beans	Apple slices with peanut butter

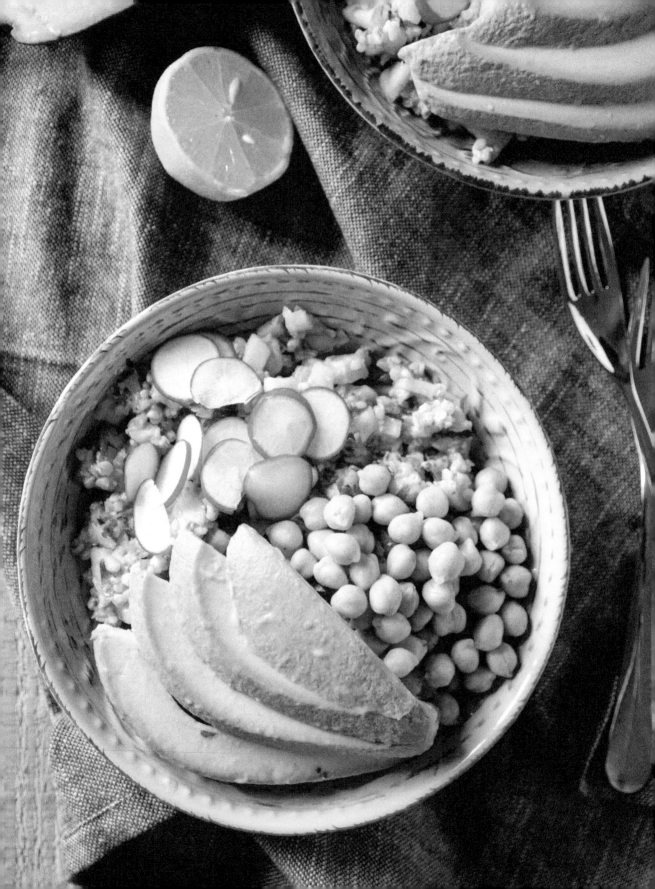

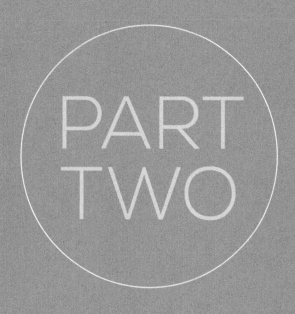

PART TWO

THE RECIPES

It's time to get cooking! Designed for success, these recipes are quick and easy to prepare without sacrificing the most important thing: taste. Enjoy the variety of meals in these chapters and start transforming your health one recipe at a time.

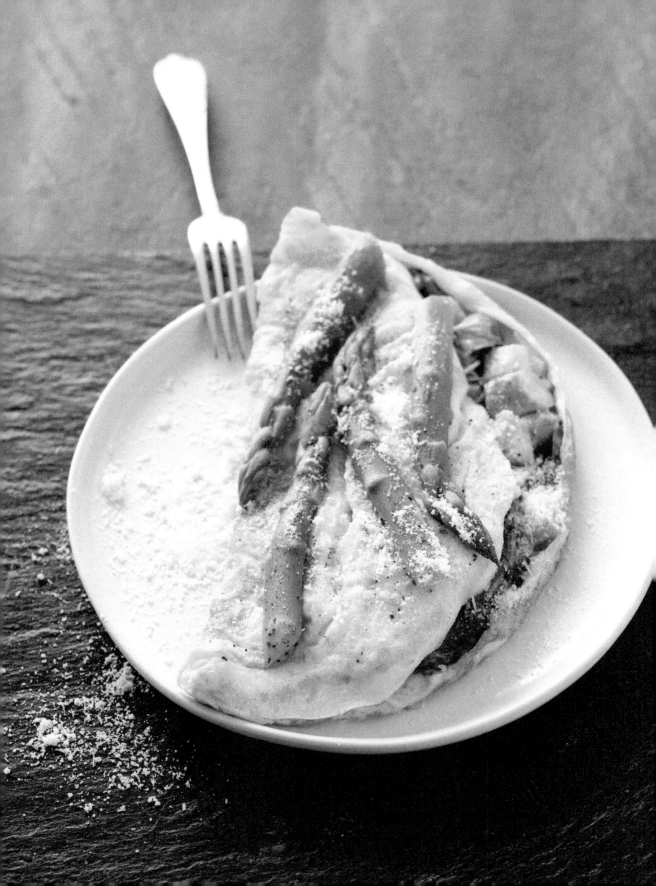

BREAKFAST &
SMOOTHIES

Starting your day with one of the filling and flavorful recipes in this chapter will help energize and nourish your body. From smoothies to scrambles, this chapter has something that will appeal to every mood and season. You'll be running out the door feeling great.

GREEN BREAKFAST SMOOTHIE

VEGETARIAN | GRAIN-FREE | GLUTEN-FREE | NUT-FREE | SOY-FREE |
KID-FRIENDLY | LOW-FODMAP

This simple smoothie is packed with protein to fill you up and takes only minutes to prepare. The banana provides a smooth texture as well as potassium, vitamin C, and vitamin B_6 for energy, while the spinach lends a pretty green hue along with folic acid, vitamin K, and carotenes. Because commercially grown spinach contains high amounts of pesticide residue, always choose organic spinach if you can.

SERVES 2

Prep time: 5 minutes

4 cups fresh baby spinach
1 large banana
1 cup ice cubes
¼ cup plain yogurt (not fat-free)
¼ cup chia seeds

Substitution Tip: If you are lactose intolerant, use dairy-free yogurt (such as coconut yogurt) or lactose-free yogurt. Goat's milk yogurt is also a good alternative, if tolerated.

In a blender, combine the spinach, banana, ice cubes, yogurt, and chia seeds. Blend until smooth. Divide evenly between two glasses and serve.

PER SERVING: Calories: 108, Protein: 5g, Cholesterol: 2mg, Sodium: 69mg, Total Carbohydrates: 19g, Fiber: 9g, Total Fat: 4g, Saturated Fat: <1g

BLUEBERRY-MELON SMOOTHIE

VEGAN | DAIRY-FREE | GRAIN-FREE | GLUTEN-FREE | NUT-FREE |
SOY-FREE | KID-FRIENDLY | LOW-FODMAP

Blueberries and melon combine in this lightly sweet and flavorful smoothie. Melons are a cooling fruit, loaded with beta-carotene and potassium, and because they are more than 90 percent water, they are extremely hydrating. Peel and dice the cantaloupe the night before and freeze it in portion-controlled containers so it is ready to go in the morning.

SERVES 1

Prep time: 5 minutes

2 cups frozen cubed
   cantaloupe melon
1 cup fresh blueberries
8 ounces water
Juice of 1 lime

Time-Saving Tip: If you know you have busy mornings ahead, make smoothies several days in advance, and freeze them in airtight containers. The night before you want it for breakfast, simply place the smoothie in the refrigerator so it is thawed by morning.

In a blender, combine the melon, blueberries, water, and lime juice. Blend until smooth. Divide evenly between two glasses and serve.

PER SERVING: Calories: 209, Protein: 4g, Cholesterol: 0mg, Sodium: 52mg, Total Carbohydrates: 54g, Fiber: 8g, Total Fat: 1g, Saturated Fat: 0g

ALMOND-BANANA SMOOTHIE

VEGETARIAN | GLUTEN-FREE | SOY-FREE | LOW-FODMAP

If you like the rich taste of almonds, you'll savor this simple blend. Almonds are a good source of protein, while the avocado adds a silky texture and provides monounsaturated fats, vitamin E, and fiber—a perfect jump-start to your day.

SERVES 2

Prep time: 5 minutes

1 frozen peeled banana

½ cup ice cubes

½ cup unsweetened rice milk, coconut milk, or nut milk

¼ avocado, chopped

¼ cup almond butter

¼ cup plain yogurt (not fat-free)

Ingredient Tip: To prevent leftover avocado from browning, sprinkle the cut side with lemon juice or lime juice, place in an airtight container, and refrigerate until ready to use. Leftover avocado will keep for a couple days.

In a blender, combine the banana, ice cubes, rice milk, avocado, almond butter, and yogurt. Blend until smooth. Divide evenly between two glasses and serve.

PER SERVING: Calories: 354, Protein: 10g, Cholesterol: 2mg, Sodium: 45mg, Total Carbohydrates: 30g, Fiber: 4g, Total Fat: 24g, Saturated Fat: 3g

FRUITY YOGURT, NUT & SEED PARFAITS

VEGETARIAN | GRAIN-FREE | GLUTEN-FREE | SOY-FREE | KID-FRIENDLY | LOW-FODMAP

These parfaits can be prepared ahead of time and kept refrigerated for up to five days, making them a good choice when you are strapped for time. Prepare these for your whole family or simply as a quick go-to for the week ahead. Packed with protein from nuts, chia seeds, and yogurt, this breakfast is at once light and filling.

SERVES 4

Prep time: 5 minutes

4 cups plain yogurt (not fat-free), divided

2 tablespoons pure maple syrup

1 teaspoon pure vanilla extract

½ cup unsalted walnuts, coarsely chopped

¼ cup chia seeds

⅛ teaspoon sea salt

1 teaspoon ground cinnamon

2 cups fresh blueberries, raspberries, or strawberries, divided

Substitution Tip: If you are lactose intolerant, use a lactose-free cow's milk yogurt or a yogurt made from coconut milk.

1. In a medium bowl, stir together the yogurt, maple syrup, and vanilla.

2. In a small bowl, combine the walnuts, chia seeds, sea salt, and cinnamon.

3. Have ready 4 large jars or cups. In each jar, build the following layers: ½ cup of yogurt, 1½ tablespoons of the nut-seed mixture, another ½ of cup yogurt, another 1½ tablespoons of the nut-seed mixture, and finishing with ½ cup of berries.

4. Serve immediately or refrigerate covered with plastic wrap for up to 5 days.

PER SERVING: Calories: 353, Protein: 19g, Cholesterol: 15mg, Sodium: 232mg, Total Carbohydrates: 38g, Fiber: 4g, Total Fat: 13g, Saturated Fat: 3g

QUINOA, BUCKWHEAT & OAT GRANOLA

VEGAN | GLUTEN-FREE | SOY-FREE | LOW-FODMAP

Packed with gluten-free grains, quinoa, nuts, and seeds, this granola is filling and flavorful. Make a batch on the weekend and serve it with yogurt or lactose-free milk for breakfast, or snack on it throughout the day to fight between-meal hunger.

SERVES 8

Prep time: 10 minutes
Cook time: 1 hour

1 cup large-flake (old-fashioned)
    rolled oats
1 cup buckwheat groats or cereal mix
½ cup raw unsalted almonds,
    coarsely chopped
½ cup raw unsalted walnuts,
    coarsely chopped
¼ cup quinoa
¼ cup chia seeds
¼ cup raw unsalted sunflower seeds
¼ cup unsweetened shredded coconut
2 teaspoons ground ginger
1 teaspoon ground cinnamon
⅛ teaspoon sea salt
¼ cup pure maple syrup
¼ cup coconut oil, melted

1. Preheat the oven to 225°F.

2. Line a large baking sheet with parchment paper.

3. In a large bowl, stir together the oats, buckwheat groats, almonds, walnuts, quinoa, chia seeds, sunflower seeds, coconut, ginger, cinnamon, and sea salt.

4. In a measuring cup, stir together the maple syrup and coconut oil. Pour the liquids over the dry ingredients and stir well to combine.

5. Spread the mixture evenly over the prepared sheet and place it in the preheated oven. Bake for 1 hour. Remove from the oven and let cool on the sheet.

6. Break the granola into clumps and store in an airtight container at room temperature for up to 8 weeks.

PER SERVING: Calories: 321, Protein: 8g, Cholesterol: 0mg, Sodium: 36mg, Total Carbohydrates: 36g, Fiber: 6g, Total Fat: 18g, Saturated Fat: 8g

PEANUT BUTTER-CHOCOLATE BREAKFAST BARS

VEGAN | GLUTEN-FREE | SOY-FREE | KID-FRIENDLY | LOW-FODMAP

Whoever said chocolate is not for breakfast had it all wrong. These delicious bars, packed with protein and fiber, are the perfect treat to brighten any morning!

MAKES 12 BARS

Prep time: 5 minutes
Cook time: 20 minutes,
    plus 2 hours chilling

1¼ cups cooked quinoa
3 cups quick-cooking
    rolled oats, divided
½ cup dark chocolate pieces or
    carob chips
¼ cup unsalted pistachios, chopped
½ cup pure maple syrup
¼ cup peanut butter

Time-Saving Tip: After cutting the bars, transfer them to an airtight container, placing a piece of wax paper or parchment paper between the bars for easy removal; refrigerate for up to 5 days. Use leftover cooked quinoa and these will take just a few minutes to pull together.

1. Preheat the oven to 350°F.

2. Line a 9-by-13-inch baking pan with parchment paper and set aside.

3. In a large bowl, stir together the quinoa, 1½ cups oats, the chocolate, and pistachios.

4. In a blender, process the remaining 1½ cups oats into oat flour. Add this to the dry mixture and stir well.

5. In a small microwave-safe bowl, stir together the maple syrup and peanut butter. If needed, microwave the mixture for 15 seconds on high to soften and help combine the mixture. Let cool.

6. Pour the cooled maple–peanut butter mixture into the dry ingredients and stir to combine.

7. Press the mixture firmly into the bottom of the prepared pan, making sure to pack the corners and sides well.

8. Bake in the preheated oven for about 20 minutes, or until lightly browned. Remove from the oven and let cool completely before refrigerating for at least 2 hours.

9. Cut into 12 even squares and serve.

PER SERVING: Calories: 186, Protein: 5g, Cholesterol: 0mg, Sodium: 34mg, Total Carbohydrates: 30g, Fiber: 3g, Total Fat: 6g, Saturated Fat: 2g

COCONUT TEFF PORRIDGE

VEGAN | DAIRY-FREE | GLUTEN-FREE | NUT-FREE | SOY-FREE | LOW-FODMAP

If the Ethiopian grain teff, most commonly known as the cornerstone of the bread *injera*, is not on your radar, go grab a bag of this nutritional powerhouse. Rich in iron and calcium, teff is a tiny grain that makes a wonderful—and naturally gluten-free—porridge. Here, both coconut milk and coconut flakes provide natural sweetness.

SERVES 2

Prep time: 5 minutes
Cook time: 15 minutes

3½ cups water
1 cup teff grains
1 cup unsweetened coconut milk
2 tablespoons unsweetened coconut
   flakes, divided

Variation Tips: For more flavor and sweetness, add a handful of your favorite berries to the porridge, such as blueberries, strawberries, or raspberries. For a bit of crunch, add 1 tablespoon of chia seeds or flaxseed, or a small handful of chopped walnuts, almonds, or pistachios.

1. In a small saucepan over high heat, combine the water and teff and bring to a boil. Cover, reduce the heat to low, and simmer for 10 minutes, stirring occasionally, until the porridge is thickened.

2. Remove the pan from the heat and stir in the coconut milk.

3. Divide the mixture evenly between two bowls and top each with 1 tablespoon of coconut flakes.

PER SERVING: Calories: 616, Protein: 15g, Cholesterol: 0mg, Sodium: 39mg, Total Carbohydrates: 73g, Fiber: 15g, Total Fat: 31g, Saturated Fat: 27g

CREAMY MILLET PORRIDGE

VEGETARIAN | GLUTEN-FREE | NUT-FREE | SOY-FREE | LOW-FODMAP

Millet is an often-underused, naturally gluten-free grain. Here it is transformed into a creamy porridge base for countless toppings. In Phase 1, top the porridge with banana, blueberries, cantaloupe, and/or kiwi. In Phase 2, choose apples, nectarines, and/or pears.

SERVES 2

Prep time: 5 minutes
Cook time: 25 minutes

---

1 cup millet
3 cups water
½ teaspoon sea salt
1 tablespoon butter

Time-Saving Tip: You can prepare millet porridge the night before and simply reheat it in the morning. To do this, cook the porridge for only 10 minutes in step 2, so there is still some liquid left in the pot, then transfer the mixture to an airtight storage container and refrigerate. Reheat before serving.

1. In a saucepan over medium-high heat, toast the millet, stirring frequently, for about 4 minutes or until golden brown.

2. Add the water and sea salt, and bring to a boil. Reduce the heat to low, cover, and simmer for 15 minutes, or until the mixture is creamy.

3. Turn off the heat and let the millet sit for an additional 10 minutes. Stir in the butter and serve.

PER SERVING: Calories: 429, Protein: 11g, Cholesterol: 15mg, Sodium: 525mg, Total Carbohydrates: 73g, Fiber: 9g, Total Fat: 10g, Saturated Fat: 4g

STEEL-CUT OATMEAL WITH NUTS & FRUIT

VEGETARIAN | GLUTEN-FREE | SOY-FREE | LOW-FODMAP

Steel-cut oats require a little more prep time than rolled or instant oats, but it is well worth the wait: these minimally processed oats are packed with flavor and nutrients. If you are not eating this oatmeal immediately, it can be cooled and refrigerated in an airtight container for up to 1 week.

SERVES 4

Prep time: 5 minutes
Cook time: 20 to 30 minutes

3 cups water
1 cup lactose-free milk or nut milk
1 cup steel-cut oats
Sea salt
½ cup fresh blueberries, divided
½ cup unsalted walnuts, divided

Phase 2 Tip: Top the oatmeal with your favorite nuts and dried fruit. Dried apricots, dates, golden raisins, cranberries, and blueberries all taste great on oats.

1. In a medium pot over medium-high heat, combine the water, milk, oats, and a pinch of sea salt and bring to a boil. Reduce the heat to medium and simmer for 20 minutes, stirring regularly until tender (if you like your oats a little softer, cook for up to 10 minutes more, stirring frequently).

2. Divide the oatmeal evenly among 4 serving bowls and top each bowl with about 2 tablespoons each of the blueberries and walnuts.

PER SERVING: Calories: 294, Protein: 12g, Cholesterol: 5mg, Sodium: 88mg, Total Carbohydrates: 34g, Fiber: 6g, Total Fat: 13g, Saturated Fat: 2g

SAVORY STEEL-CUT OATMEAL WITH SPINACH

VEGETARIAN | GLUTEN-FREE | NUT-FREE | SOY-FREE | LOW-FODMAP

Oatmeal doesn't have to be sweet. This recipe combines spinach and Parmesan cheese with steel-cut oats for a savory spin on a classic and a burst of B vitamins to start your day right. You can make this oatmeal in advance and then simply refrigerate it and reheat in the morning for a quick meal.

SERVES 4

Prep time: 5 minutes
Cook time: 15 minutes

1¼ cups steel-cut oats
3½ cups water
1 cup packed thinly sliced
    fresh spinach
¼ cup grated Parmesan cheese

Substitution Tip: Use kale or another favorite green instead of spinach. Young collard greens, mustard greens, and arugula are all flavorful substitutions for spinach that are widely available year-round.

1. In a dry pot over medium heat, toast the oatmeal until golden brown.

2. Add the water, increase the heat to high, and bring the mixture to a boil. Reduce the heat to medium-low, cover, and simmer for 15 minutes, or until the oatmeal is tender and the water has been absorbed.

3. Add the spinach and stir until it is wilted. Add the Parmesan cheese and stir until combined. Serve.

PER SERVING: Calories: 244, Protein: 12g, Cholesterol: 10mg, Sodium: 138mg, Total Carbohydrates: 35g, Fiber: 5g, Total Fat: 6g, Saturated Fat: 3g

BLUEBERRY-COCONUT QUINOA BREAKFAST BOWL

VEGAN | DAIRY-FREE | GLUTEN-FREE | NUT | FREE | SOY-FREE | LOW-FODMAP

Move over oatmeal—quinoa is the new breakfast darling in town. Quinoa cooks into a porridge in the same amount of time as oatmeal, and the flavor combinations are just as endless. Here, coconut and blueberries create a tasty breakfast bowl packed with antioxidants and healthy fat.

SERVES 2

Prep time: 5 minutes
Cook time: 15 to 20 minutes

1 teaspoon extra virgin olive oil
¾ cup quinoa, rinsed and drained
1 (15-ounce) can reduced-fat
    unsweetened coconut milk
1 tablespoon pure maple syrup
2 tablespoons unsweetened
    shredded coconut, divided
½ cup fresh blueberries, divided
2 tablespoons chia seeds, divided

Substitution Tip: If preferred, substitute raspberries or strawberries for the blueberries.

1. In a pot over medium heat, heat the olive oil. Add the quinoa and toast, stirring constantly until it is a light golden brown color.

2. Stir in the coconut milk and bring the mixture to a boil. Reduce the heat to low, cover, and simmer for 15 to 20 minutes until the liquid is absorbed. Stir in the maple syrup.

3. Divide the porridge into 2 bowls. Top each bowl with 1 tablespoon of coconut, ¼ cup of blueberries, and 1 tablespoon of chia seeds.

PER SERVING: Calories: 622, Protein: 19g, Cholesterol: 0mg, Sodium: 60mg, Total Carbohydrates: 73g, Fiber: 17g, Total Fat: 31g, Saturated Fat: 15g

BANANA OAT PANCAKES

VEGETARIAN | GLUTEN-FREE | SOY-FREE | LOW-FODMAP

This might be one of the simplest pancake recipes out there: Toss the ingredients in the blender and—*voilà!*—you've got a batter ready to pour into a hot pan and fry into fluffy, flavorful pancakes. Bananas not only lend sweetness, but also are high in potassium, and vitamins B_6 and C.

SERVES 4

Prep time: 5 minutes
Cook time: 15 minutes

2 cups quick-cooking rolled oats
1¼ cups lactose-free milk or nut milk
1 banana
1 tablespoon pure maple syrup, plus
   additional for serving
1½ teaspoons baking powder
1 teaspoon pure vanilla extract
½ teaspoon ground cinnamon
¼ teaspoon sea salt
1 large egg
Butter, for frying

Time-Saving Tip: Pancakes freeze wonderfully. Make a double batch and freeze the extras in a freezer-safe storage bag with small pieces of parchment paper between them to make for easy separation. Unlike waffles, you can reheat pancakes in the microwave or toaster for a quick breakfast.

1. In a blender, combine the oats, milk, banana, maple syrup, baking powder, vanilla, cinnamon, and sea salt. Blend until smooth. Add the egg and pulse a few times just to combine.

2. In a large skillet over medium heat, melt 1 teaspoon of butter. Scoop ¼-cup portions of batter into the skillet. Cook for 2 to 3 minutes, until the bottoms are lightly browned and small bubbles appear on the surface of the pancakes. Using a spatula, flip the pancakes and cook on the other side for 2 to 3 minutes, or until golden brown. Transfer to a plate, keeping them warm, and repeat with the remaining butter and batter. Serve with maple syrup.

PER SERVING: Calories: 256, Protein: 10g, Cholesterol: 53mg, Sodium: 175mg, Total Carbohydrates: 43g, Fiber: 5g, Total Fat: 6g, Saturated Fat: 2g

BUCKWHEAT PANCAKES WITH BLUEBERRY SYRUP

VEGETARIAN | GLUTEN-FREE | NUT-FREE | SOY-FREE | LOW-FODMAP

These buckwheat pancakes are light and airy, with a slightly nutty flavor thanks to the buckwheat. Lysine, an important amino acid, is contained in buckwheat's black hull, so choose dark varieties of buckwheat flour for the most nutrition.

SERVES 4

Prep time: 10 minutes
Cook time: 20 minutes

For the blueberry sauce
1 cup fresh blueberries
¼ cup pure maple syrup

For the pancakes
1½ cups buckwheat flour
1 teaspoon baking powder
½ teaspoon ground cinnamon
⅛ teaspoon sea salt
1 large egg
¾ cup unsweetened rice milk, coconut milk, or nut milk
2 tablespoons butter

Substitution Tip: If you are a vegan or intolerant of egg, you can substitute 1 tablespoon of ground chia seeds or flaxseed soaked in 3 tablespoons of water for the egg. Let the mixture soak for 2 to 5 minutes, until the water is mostly absorbed. You can also substitute coconut oil for the butter and proceed with the recipe.

To make the blueberry syrup

In a blender, combine the blueberries and maple syrup and blend until just combined (it should still be a little chunky). Set aside.

To make the pancakes

1. In a large bowl, whisk together the flour, baking powder, cinnamon, and sea salt.

2. In another bowl whisk together the egg and milk. Gradually pour the wet ingredients into the dry ingredients, whisking until a smooth batter is formed.

3. Place a large frying pan over medium-high heat. Rub the pan with butter to coat. Ladle enough batter into the pan to make 3- to 4-inch pancakes. Fry for 3 to 4 minutes, until tiny bubbles appear on the surface. Using a spatula, flip the pancakes and cook on other side for 3 to 4 minutes until browned. Transfer to a plate, and repeat with the remaining batter. Serve warm topped with blueberry syrup.

PER SERVING: Calories: 302, Protein: 8g, Cholesterol: 62mg, Sodium: 150mg, Total Carbohydrates: 53g, Fiber: 7g, Total Fat: 9g, Saturated Fat: 4g

BUCKWHEAT CRÊPES WITH SOUTHWESTERN SCRAMBLE

VEGETARIAN | GLUTEN-FREE | SOY-FREE

Crêpes are a light and airy foundation for all sorts of savory and sweet fillings. Made with buckwheat flour, these crêpes have a slightly nutty flavor that marries perfectly with a Southwestern-inspired scramble.

SERVES 4

Prep time: 5 minutes
Cook time: 15 minutes

---

6 large eggs, divided
½ cup almond milk
⅓ cup buckwheat flour
5 teaspoons coconut oil, divided
Sea salt
Freshly ground black pepper
½ cup tomato salsa, plus additional for serving
½ cup shredded Cheddar cheese

Substitution Tip: The variations on this recipe are only limited by your imagination. Try a feta and spinach scramble, or even a kimchi and egg scramble.

1. In a large bowl, whisk together 2 eggs, the almond milk, and buckwheat flour.

2. Heat a large skillet over medium-high heat. Add 1 teaspoon of coconut oil and swirl to coat the pan. Drop ¼-cup portions of batter into the skillet, swirling to cover the bottom of the pan in a light coating of batter. Cook for about 1 minute until the edges are crisp. Flip and cook for 30 seconds more. Transfer to a plate, keeping warm, and repeat with 3 teaspoons of coconut oil and batter to make a total of 4 crêpes.

3. In the same skillet over medium-high heat, melt the remaining 1 teaspoon of coconut oil. Add the remaining 4 eggs and season to taste with sea salt and pepper. Cook just until the bottom of the eggs begins to set, then, using a spatula, scramble them. When the eggs are nearly set, add the salsa and Cheddar cheese. Stir together and cook until the eggs are done to your liking.

4. Divide the eggs evenly among the 4 crêpes and serve topped with additional salsa.

PER SERVING: Calories: 324, Protein: 15g, Cholesterol: 294mg, Sodium: 452mg, Total Carbohydrates: 11g, Fiber: 2g, Total Fat: 25g, Saturated Fat: 17g

OATMEAL WAFFLES

VEGETARIAN | GLUTEN-FREE | SOY-FREE | LOW-FODMAP

Don't think you have to give up waffles just because you are avoiding gluten during Phase 1. These simple oatmeal waffles, with their crisp exterior and fluffy interior, rival any wheat-based versions. You will need a blender to make the oat flour. If you are gluten intolerant, use certified gluten-free oats.

SERVES 4

Prep time: 20 minutes
Cook time: 30 minutes

1½ cups quick-cooking rolled oats
2 teaspoons baking powder
½ teaspoon sea salt
2 large eggs
1 cup lactose-free milk or nut milk
5 tablespoons butter, melted
1 teaspoon pure vanilla extract

Time-Saving Tip: Waffles freeze well. Make a double batch and freeze half in a freezer-safe bag. When you want one for breakfast, simply pop it in the toaster.

1. In a blender, process the oats until they resemble a fine flour.

2. In a large bowl, combine the oat flour, baking powder, and sea salt and stir well.

3. In another bowl or measuring cup, whisk together the eggs, milk, butter, and vanilla. Fold the wet ingredients into the dry ingredients and stir until just combined (just make sure all the dry ingredients are incorporated). Set aside for 10 minutes to rest.

4. Preheat the oven to 200°F.

5. Heat a waffle iron according to the manufacturer's instructions.

6. Stir the batter after resting. Scoop about ⅓ cup of batter into the waffle iron, using the back of the cup to spread the batter on the iron. Close the waffle iron and cook for 4 to 6 minutes until the waffle is golden brown and crisp (the exact time will depend on your waffle iron). Transfer the cooked waffles to the warm oven, arranging them in a single layer (avoid stacking the waffles, as this can cause them to become soggy), and repeat until the batter is used up.

PER SERVING: Calories: 315, Protein: 9g, Cholesterol: 136mg, Sodium: 404mg, Total Carbohydrates: 25g, Fiber: 3g, Total Fat: 20g, Saturated Fat: 11g

PARMESAN-BASIL SCRAMBLED EGGS

VEGETARIAN | GRAIN-FREE | GLUTEN-FREE | NUT-FREE | SOY-FREE | LOW-FODMAP

This Italian-inspired scramble, full of brightly flavored basil, is loaded with protein to keep you feeling full all morning. If you don't have fresh basil, substitute dried basil and reduce the amount by half.

SERVES 2

Prep time: 5 minutes
Cook time: 10 minutes

4 large eggs

¼ teaspoon sea salt

¼ teaspoon freshly ground
  black pepper

1 teaspoon extra virgin olive oil

2 tablespoons finely chopped fresh
  basil or 1 tablespoon dried basil

2 tablespoons grated
  Parmesan cheese

Variation Tip: Try this scramble with sharp Cheddar cheese instead of Parmesan cheese. You can also substitute an equal amount of cilantro for the basil.

1. In a small bowl, whisk together the eggs, sea salt, and pepper.

2. In a small skillet over medium-high heat, heat the olive oil. Add the beaten eggs and cook for 30 to 45 seconds, just until they begin to set. Using a spatula, stir the eggs in a swirling motion. Reduce the heat to medium-low and cook, stirring constantly until the eggs are nearly set. Stir in the basil and Parmesan cheese.

3. When the eggs are done to your liking, remove the pan from the heat. Divide the eggs between 2 plates and serve immediately.

PER SERVING: Calories: 254, Protein: 22g, Cholesterol: 392mg, Sodium: 634mg, Total Carbohydrates: 2g, Fiber: 0g, Total Fat: 18g, Saturated Fat: 7g

MISO SCRAMBLED EGGS

VEGETARIAN | DAIRY-FREE | NUT-FREE

The salty flavor of fermented miso adds a tasty complexity to this simple-to-prepare dish. Don't be tempted to add the miso while the eggs are still cooking, or you'll negate their probiotic benefit, which is killed in the cooking process.

SERVES 2

Prep time: 5 minutes
Cook time: 10 minutes

4 large eggs
¼ teaspoon freshly ground
   black pepper
1 teaspoon extra virgin olive oil
2 tablespoons red miso paste or
   white miso paste

Ingredient Tip: White miso is generally milder than red, which is more robustly flavored. Look for miso that is unpasteurized and naturally fermented, as some brands use chemicals to ferment their soy. If soy is an allergen, choose miso made from chickpeas, which you can find at natural food stores.

1. In a small bowl, whisk together the eggs and pepper.

2. In a large skillet over medium-high heat, heat the olive oil. Add the beaten eggs and cook for 30 to 45 seconds, just until they begin to set on the bottom. Using a spatula, stir the eggs in a swirling motion. Reduce the heat to low and cook, stirring constantly until the eggs are done to your liking. Remove the pan from the heat.

3. Add the miso and stir until well combined. Divide the eggs between 2 plates and serve immediately.

PER SERVING: Calories: 198, Protein: 15g, Cholesterol: 372mg, Sodium: 781mg, Total Carbohydrates: 6g, Fiber: 1g, Total Fat: 13g, Saturated Fat: 4g

FETA & SPINACH OMELET

VEGETARIAN | GRAIN-FREE | GLUTEN-FREE | NUT-FREE | SOY-FREE | LOW-FODMAP

Feta and spinach pair wonderfully in this Greek-inspired omelet. Because feta cheese is rather salty, there is no need to add additional salt. Goat's milk feta is often tolerated by people who are lactose intolerant.

SERVES 2

Prep time: 5 minutes
Cook time: 10 minutes

---

4 large eggs
¼ teaspoon freshly ground black pepper
1 teaspoon extra virgin olive oil
¼ cup feta cheese
2 cups fresh baby spinach

Phase 2 Tip: Top the omelet with 4 to 6 spears of roasted or steamed asparagus and a generous sprinkling of Parmesan cheese.

Ingredient Tip: When buying feta cheese, save money by buying bricks of feta and crumbling it yourself. A bonus: Whole feta stores longer in the refrigerator.

1. In a small bowl, whisk together the eggs and pepper.

2. In a small skillet over medium heat, heat the olive oil. Add the beaten eggs and cook for about 3 minutes until the bottom is well set, but the top is still runny.

3. Evenly sprinkle the feta cheese over half of the omelet. Top the feta with the spinach, pushing it down gently with a spatula to hold it in place. Using the spatula, fold the uncovered half of the omelet over the spinach. Cook for about 1 minute, then carefully flip the whole omelet. Cook for 2 to 3 minutes more until the middle is set.

4. To serve, divide the omelet evenly between 2 plates.

PER SERVING: Calories: 220, Protein: 16g, Cholesterol: 389mg, Sodium: 373mg, Total Carbohydrates: 3g, Fiber: <1g, Total Fat: 16g, Saturated Fat: 6g

KIMCHI OMELET

VEGETARIAN | GRAIN-FREE | GLUTEN-FREE | NUT-FREE | SOY-FREE | LOW-FODMAP

Make your own Kimchi (page 245) or choose your favorite purchased version for this simple and filling Asian-inspired omelet. How much salt you add will depend on how salty your kimchi is, so taste it before seasoning this dish further.

SERVES 2

Prep time: 5 minutes
Cook time: 10 minutes

---

4 large eggs
1 teaspoon rice wine vinegar
¼ teaspoon freshly ground
    black pepper
Sea salt
1 teaspoon extra virgin olive oil
2 scallions (green part only),
    thinly sliced
¼ cup chopped kimchi
2 tablespoons shredded
    Cheddar cheese

Phase 1 Tip: To make this recipe a good choice for Phase 1, make it using the Kimchi on page 245. Some brands of purchased kimchi contain large amounts of garlic, which should be avoided during Phase 1 of the diet.

1. In a small bowl, whisk together the eggs, rice wine vinegar, and pepper. Season to taste with sea salt.

2. In a small skillet over medium heat, heat the olive oil. Add the scallion greens and kimchi and cook, stirring constantly until heated through.

3. Add the egg mixture and cook for 2 minutes, or until the bottom is well set but the top is still runny. Evenly sprinkle the Cheddar over one-half of the omelet. Using a spatula, fold the uncovered half of the omelet over the cheese. Cook for 1 to 2 minutes, then carefully flip the whole omelet. Cook for 2 to 3 minutes more until the middle is set.

4. To serve, divide the omelet evenly between 2 plates.

PER SERVING: Calories: 206, Protein: 15g, Cholesterol: 379mg, Sodium: 421mg, Total Carbohydrates: 3g, Fiber: 1g, Total Fat: 15g, Saturated Fat: 5g

EGGS "BENEKRAUT"

VEGETARIAN | NUT-FREE | LOW-FODMAP

Vegetables for breakfast? Absolutely. This twist on traditional eggs Benedict features creamy avocado and tangy cultured sauerkraut. Rich hollandaise sauce tops off this satisfying morning meal.

SERVES 2

Prep time: 20 minutes
Cook time: 25 minutes

For the eggs "Benekraut"

4 slices spelt bread (or other low-FODMAP bread)
¼ cup fermented Sauerkraut (page 242), divided
¼ avocado, sliced, divided
1 tablespoon white vinegar
4 medium eggs

For the hollandaise sauce

4 medium egg yolks
1 tablespoon fresh lemon juice
½ cup butter, melted
¼ teaspoon smoked paprika

To make the eggs "Benekraut"

1. Using the top of a wide glass, cut a round from the center of each slice of bread. Arrange two rounds on each plate.

2. Top each bread round with sauerkraut and avocado.

3. Fill a medium saucepan with 4 inches of water and bring to a gentle simmer. Stir in the vinegar.

4. Working with one egg at a time, carefully crack the egg into the simmering water and immediately lift the pot and swirl the water gently in one direction. Place the pot back on the burner and poach the egg for about 4 minutes. Using a slotted spoon, transfer the poached egg to a plate lined with paper towel. Repeat with the remaining eggs.

5. To serve, place a poached egg on top of each round and top each egg with hollandaise.

To make the hollandaise sauce

1. In a small saucepan, vigorously whisk together the egg yolks and lemon juice for 1 to 2 minutes until thickened and doubled in volume.

2. Place the saucepan over low heat. Whisk in the melted butter and cook for 5 to 7 minutes, stirring constantly until the mixture is slightly thickened. Add the paprika and whisk to combine.

3. Pour the hollandaise sauce over each serving of eggs "Benekraut" and serve immediately.

PER SERVING: Calories: 899, Protein: 24g, Cholesterol: 869mg, Sodium: 967mg, Total Carbohydrates: 48g, Fiber: 4g, Total Fat: 71g, Saturated Fat: 36g

Cooking Tip: To make poaching an egg easier, crack the egg onto a rimless dessert plate or into a small cup, taking care not to pierce the yolk, then gently slide the egg into the simmering water.

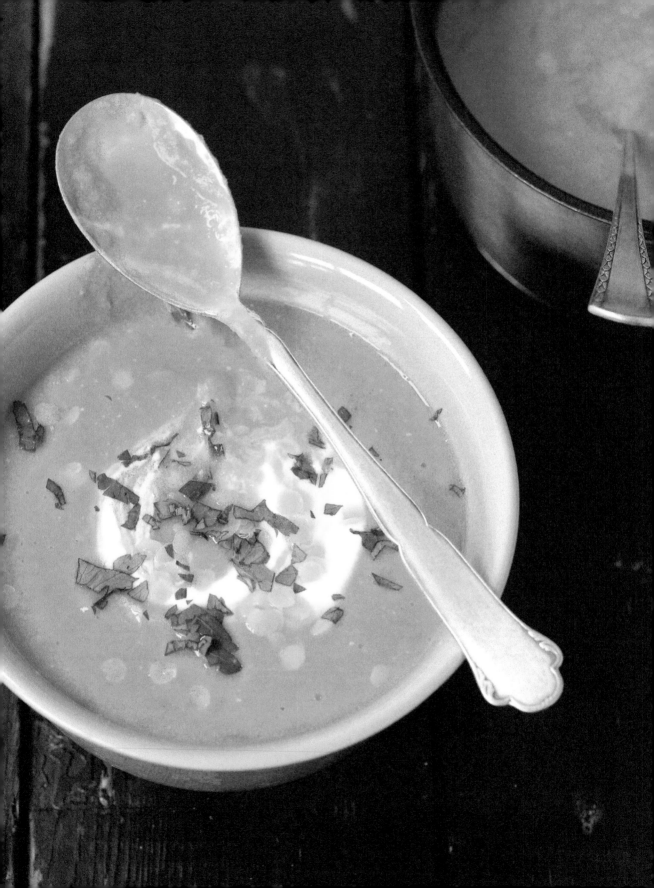

SOUPS & SALADS

There is nothing more comforting than a warm bowl of soup. All your favorites are here, reworked to support your health in both phases of the Microbiome Diet. Whether you like a creamy or stock-based soup, there is something here for you. There are also plenty of fresh green and fruit salads to accompany these soups for a light lunch or dinner.

VEGETABLE STOCK

VEGAN | DAIRY-FREE | GRAIN-FREE | GLUTEN-FREE | NUT-FREE |
SOY-FREE | KID-FRIENDLY | LOW-FODMAP

This simple but nourishing stock is the building block of many recipes in this chapter. Make it on a weekend afternoon and you'll be well equipped for the week ahead. Feel free to add other favorite chopped vegetables, or even vegetable scraps, to this recipe, but be sure to adhere to the vegetables listed in the chart on pages 45 and 47 for each phase.

MAKES 12 CUPS STOCK

Prep time: 10 minutes
Cook time: 50 minutes,
   plus 30 minutes cooling

2 tablespoons extra virgin olive oil
1 head fennel, roughly chopped
1 bunch leeks (green part only)
6 carrots, roughly chopped
16 cups water
1 bunch scallions
   (green part only)
½ bunch fresh flat-leaf Italian parsley
2 bay leaves
1 teaspoon whole black peppercorns
1 teaspoon sea salt

*Phase 2 Tip: Once you are in
Phase 2, you can add several cloves
of garlic and 1 large diced onion
in step 1 for even more flavor.
If adding the onion, omit the
scallion greens.*

1. In a large stockpot over medium-high heat, heat the olive oil until it shimmers. Add the fennel, leeks, and carrots. Cook for about 5 minutes, stirring frequently until the vegetables are near tender.

2. Add the water, scallion greens, parsley, bay leaves, peppercorns, and sea salt and bring to a boil. Reduce the heat to low and simmer, partially covered, for 45 minutes.

3. Pour the stock through a fine-mesh strainer into a large pot, pressing on the vegetables with the back of a large spoon to extract as much liquid as possible. Discard the solids. Let the stock cool for about 30 minutes, and then transfer it to 2-cup airtight containers and freeze until needed.

PER SERVING: Calories: 38, Protein: 5g, Cholesterol: 0mg, Sodium: 763mg, Total Carbohydrates: 1g, Fiber: 0g, Total Fat: 0g, Saturated Fat: 0g

CHICKEN STOCK

DAIRY-FREE | GRAIN-FREE | GLUTEN-FREE | NUT-FREE | SOY-FREE |
KID-FRIENDLY | LOW-FODMAP

Finding a prepared chicken stock that is both gluten-free and doesn't contain garlic and onion is a nearly impossible task (there are a few brands, but they can be difficult to find). The good news is that it is pretty simple to make, and, when you use this recipe that starts with a whole chicken, you end up with a sizable amount of cooked meat for other chicken entrées.

MAKES 10 CUPS STOCK

Prep time: 10 minutes
Cook time: 1 hour, 40 minutes,
   plus cooling time

---

1 whole (2- to 3-pound) chicken,
   cut into 8 pieces
16 cups water
3 bay leaves
2 carrots, roughly chopped
½ bunch fresh flat-leaf Italian parsley
1 teaspoon whole black peppercorns
½ teaspoon dried oregano

Phase 2 Tip: Once you are in Phase 2, you can add several cloves of garlic and 1 large diced onion in step 1 for even more flavor.

1. In a large stockpot over high heat, combine the chicken, water, bay leaves, carrots, parsley, peppercorns, and oregano, and bring to a boil. Using a spoon, skim off and discard any scum that rises to the top. Reduce the heat to low and simmer for about 40 minutes until the chicken pieces are cooked through.

2. Using tongs or a slotted spoon, transfer the chicken pieces to a colander set over a bowl and let drain. When the chicken is cool enough to handle, pick the meat from the bones and set aside; discard the skin and return the bones to the stockpot. Chop the meat into bite-size pieces and package in 2-cup containers; freeze or refrigerate as needed for future meals. Continue to simmer the stock for 1 hour more.

3. Using a fine-mesh strainer, strain the bones, vegetables, and herbs from the stock into a clean bowl. You should be left with about 10 cups of stock. Divide the stock into 1- or 2-cup portions and set aside until completely cool. Cover and refrigerate for up to 5 days, or freeze for up to 1 year.

PER SERVING: Calories: 38, Protein: 5g, Cholesterol: 0mg, Sodium: 763mg, Total Carbohydrates: 1g, Fiber: 0g, Total Fat: 1g, Saturated Fat: 0g

PUMPKIN SOUP

VEGETARIAN | GRAIN-FREE | GLUTEN-FREE | NUT-FREE | SOY-FREE | LOW-FODMAP

Pumpkin isn't just for pies. The lightly sweet winter squash also makes a splendid, delicately spiced soup. Use canned pure pumpkin purée and this robust soup will be ready to eat in about 20 minutes from start to finish.

SERVES 4

Prep time: 5 minutes
Cook time: 10 minutes

1 tablespoon butter
Pinch asafetida
2 cups Vegetable Stock (page 99)
1 (15-ounce) can pure pumpkin purée
1 cup unsweetened coconut milk
2 tablespoons pure maple syrup
¼ teaspoon freshly ground
    black pepper
¼ teaspoon ground nutmeg
¼ teaspoon ground cinnamon
Sea salt

Cooking Tip: If you don't have an immersion blender, simply transfer the soup to a standard blender and purée in batches.

1. In a large saucepan over medium-high heat, melt the butter. Add the asafetida and cook for about 15 seconds, stirring constantly until fragrant. Stir in the vegetable stock, pumpkin, coconut milk, maple syrup, pepper, nutmeg, and cinnamon. Season to taste with sea salt. Bring to a boil, reduce the heat to low, and simmer for 5 to 10 minutes.

2. Using an immersion blender, purée the soup. Serve.

PER SERVING: Calories: 254, Protein: 6g, Cholesterol: 8mg, Sodium: 479mg, Total Carbohydrates: 21g, Fiber: 4g, Total Fat: 18g, Saturated Fat: 15g

CREAMY AVOCADO SOUP

VEGETARIAN | GRAIN-FREE | GLUTEN-FREE | NUT-FREE | SOY-FREE | LOW-FODMAP

Avocado makes a wonderfully creamy soup with a rich color and flavor. Best when served cold, this simple soup is loaded with healthy fats from the avocado and olive oil, and a heaping dose of nutrients from the spinach and tomatoes. Prepare this in advance so it has plenty of time to chill before serving.

SERVES 4

Prep time: 15 minutes
Cook time: 10 minutes

1 large ripe avocado,
    pitted and peeled
2 tablespoons fresh lemon juice
1 tablespoon extra virgin olive oil
Pinch asafetida
2 tomatoes, seeded
2 cups fresh baby spinach
1 small red chile pepper
2 cups Vegetable Stock (page 99)
⅔ cup lactose-free milk or nut milk

Variation Tip: If you like, garnish the soup with a couple tablespoons of shredded Cheddar cheese or crumbled feta cheese before serving.

1. Place the avocado in a bowl and mash with a fork. Add the lemon juice and stir well to combine. Set aside.

2. In a skillet over medium-high heat, heat the olive oil. Add the asafetida and cook for about 10 seconds, stirring until fragrant.

3. Add the tomatoes, spinach, and chile pepper. Sauté for 2 to 3 minutes. Remove the pan from the heat.

4. Transfer half of the tomato mixture to a blender and purée until smooth. Add the mashed avocado and blend until smooth.

5. Transfer the blended mixture to a clean pot over low heat. Stir in the remaining tomato mixture, vegetable stock, and milk. Cook, stirring occasionally until just heated through. Serve immediately, or refrigerate for at least 2 hours to serve cold.

PER SERVING: Calories: 189, Protein: 6g, Cholesterol: 3mg, Sodium: 420mg, Total Carbohydrates: 10g, Fiber: 5g, Total Fat: 15g, Saturated Fat: 3g

BROCCOLI & SPINACH CHEDDAR SOUP

VEGETARIAN | GRAIN-FREE | GLUTEN-FREE | NUT-FREE | SOY-FREE |
KID-FRIENDLY | LOW-FODMAP

This filling soup packs a serious broccoli and spinach punch. Unlike most cream of broccoli soups thickened with milk, this version uses Cheddar cheese for creaminess and whole-grain mustard for added flavor.

SERVES 4

Prep time: 5 minutes
Cook time: 15 minutes

1 tablespoon extra virgin olive oil
Pinch asafetida
4 cups Vegetable Stock (page 99)
4 cups fresh baby spinach
2 cups broccoli florets
1 teaspoon sea salt
1 tablespoon whole-grain mustard
1 cup shredded Cheddar cheese

Phase 2 Tip: Once in Phase 2, you can make this soup entirely with broccoli. Omit the spinach and add 2 more cups of broccoli, for a total of 4 cups. For a heartier soup, add 1 or 2 diced, peeled potatoes along with the broccoli.

1. In a large saucepan over medium-high heat, heat the olive oil. Add the asafetida and cook for about 15 seconds, stirring constantly until fragrant. Add the vegetable stock, spinach, broccoli, and sea salt and bring to a boil. Reduce the heat to low and simmer for 5 to 10 minutes until the broccoli is just tender. Using an immersion blender, purée the soup.

2. Stir in the mustard. Add the Cheddar cheese and stir to combine. Taste and adjust the seasoning, if desired.

PER SERVING: Calories: 212, Protein: 14g, Cholesterol: 30mg, Sodium: 1,446mg, Total Carbohydrates: 6g, Fiber: 2g, Total Fat: 15g, Saturated Fat: 7g

CREAMY TOMATO & SPINACH SOUP

VEGETARIAN | GRAIN-FREE | GLUTEN-FREE | NUT-FREE | SOY-FREE | KID-FRIENDLY | LOW-FODMAP

Tomato soup is a fantastic comfort food, and there is no reason to leave it behind on the Microbiome Diet. Forget about the stuff from a can, which is loaded with preservatives, and follow this simple recipe to make a tasty soup with next to no effort.

SERVES 4

Prep time: 5 minutes
Cook time: 15 minutes

1 tablespoon butter
Pinch asafetida
2 (15-ounce) cans diced tomatoes
　　with juices
1 (6-ounce) can tomato paste
1 cup Vegetable Stock (page 99)
　　or water
2 cups unsweetened coconut milk
4 cups fresh baby spinach
Sea salt
Freshly ground black pepper

Phase 2 Tip: If preferred, substitute 1 finely chopped onion for the asafetida in step 1. Sauté the onion until softened before adding the tomatoes and other ingredients. You can also chop up 2 celery stalks and add them to the soup in step 1.

1. In a large saucepan over medium-high heat, melt the butter. Add the asafetida and cook for about 15 seconds, stirring constantly until fragrant. Add the tomatoes, tomato paste, and vegetable stock and bring to a boil. Reduce the heat to low and simmer for 5 minutes.

2. Remove the pan from the heat and, using an immersion blender, purée the soup. Return the pan to the heat. Stir in the coconut milk and bring the mixture to a simmer. Cook for 5 minutes.

3. Add the spinach and stir constantly until wilted. Season to taste with sea salt and pepper. Serve.

PER SERVING: Calories: 391, Protein: 9g, Cholesterol: 8mg, Sodium: 363mg, Total Carbohydrates: 24g, Fiber: 8g, Total Fat: 33g, Saturated Fat: 27g

BLACK BEAN SOUP

VEGAN | DAIRY-FREE | GRAIN-FREE | GLUTEN-FREE | NUT-FREE | SOY-FREE

Black bean soup is very quick to make when using canned beans, and tastes like it's been simmering all day. Using cumin as its standout seasoning, this soup is filling, nourishing, and loaded with fiber. Enjoy on its own, or serve it topped with a little plain yogurt, with a side of hot white or brown rice.

SERVES 4

Prep time: 5 minutes
Cook time: 15 minutes

---

1 tablespoon extra virgin olive oil
Pinch asafetida
1 green bell pepper, diced
3 cups Vegetable Stock (page 99)
2 (15-ounce) cans black beans,
    rinsed and drained
1 teaspoon sea salt
½ teaspoon freshly ground black
    pepper
½ teaspoon ground cumin
2 tablespoons white vinegar
Chopped scallions (green part only),
    for garnish

Ingredient Tip: To cook your own black beans for this recipe, place 1 cup dried beans in a pot and cover with several inches of cold water. Set aside to soak overnight. Then drain the water and cover the beans with about 2 inches of fresh water. Bring to boil. Cover, reduce the heat to low, and simmer the beans for 30 to 45 minutes until tender. While you are at it, make extra and freeze them, covered in their cooking liquid, in 2-cup portions for later use.

1. In a large saucepan over medium-high heat, heat the olive oil. Add the asafetida and cook for about 15 seconds, stirring constantly until fragrant. Add the green bell pepper and cook, stirring constantly until just beginning to soften. Stir in the vegetable stock, black beans, sea salt, pepper, and cumin and bring to a boil. Cover, reduce the heat to low, and simmer for 15 minutes.

2. Using a potato masher, gently mash about half of the beans in the pot.

3. Stir in the white vinegar. Taste and adjust the seasonings, if desired. Serve garnished with the scallion greens.

PER SERVING: Calories: 796, Protein: 50g, Cholesterol: 0mg, Sodium: 1,053mg, Total Carbohydrates: 135g, Fiber: 33g, Total Fat: 8g, Saturated Fat: 2g

LENTIL-CARROT SOUP

VEGAN | DAIRY-FREE | GLUTEN-FREE | NUT-FREE | SOY-FREE

A healthy dose of carrots lends sweetness to this earthy red lentil soup that is blended until creamy—a comforting alternative to traditional lentil soup.

SERVES 4

Prep time: 5 minutes
Cook time: 35 minutes

6 medium carrots, roughly chopped
4 cups Vegetable Stock (page 99)
1 (8-ounce) can tomato sauce
¾ cup dried red lentils
Pinch asafetida
1 tablespoon extra virgin olive oil
1 teaspoon ground cumin
1 teaspoon ground coriander
½ teaspoon ground turmeric
½ teaspoon cayenne pepper
1 tablespoon fresh lemon juice
1¼ cups unsweetened coconut milk
Sea salt

Variation Tip: Spoon a bit of yogurt into each bowl when serving. Not only will this lend rich flavor, but it is also a great probiotic punch. Top with a bit of basil chiffonade for a touch of freshness and color.

1. In a large saucepan over medium-high heat, combine the carrots, vegetable stock, tomato sauce, lentils, and asafetida and bring to a boil. Cover, reduce the heat to low, and simmer for 30 minutes, or until the lentils are tender.

2. Remove the pot from the heat and, using an immersion blender, purée the soup.

3. In a small skillet over medium heat, heat the olive oil. Stir in the cumin, coriander, turmeric, and cayenne pepper. Cook for about 1 minute, stirring constantly until just fragrant. Remove from the heat. Stir in the lemon juice.

4. Immediately pour the spice mixture into the soup pot, using a spatula to scrape in as much as possible. Stir in the coconut milk.

5. Place the soup over medium heat and cook just until heated through. Season to taste with sea salt and serve.

PER SERVING: Calories: 424, Protein: 18g, Cholesterol: 0mg, Sodium: 1,139mg, Total Carbohydrates: 39g, Fiber: 16g, Total Fat: 23g, Saturated Fat: 17g

CHICKEN VEGETABLE SOUP

DAIRY-FREE | GLUTEN-FREE | NUT-FREE | SOY-FREE | KID-FRIENDLY | LOW-FODMAP

Bursting with rich flavor thanks to the chicken, this soup is a weekday winner. Save any leftovers for easy lunches, or double the recipe and freeze the extra portions to have on hand when cooking is not an option.

SERVES 4

Prep time: 10 minutes
Cook time: 30 minutes

1 tablespoon extra virgin olive oil
3 carrots, halved lengthwise
    and chopped
2 small zucchini, halved lengthwise
    and chopped
1 red bell pepper, seeded and diced
1 leek (green part only), chopped
5 cups Chicken Stock (page 100)
1 tomato, diced
¼ cup finely chopped fresh flat-leaf
    Italian parsley
2 sprigs fresh thyme
1 bay leaf
2 cups cooked chicken
Sea salt
Freshly ground black pepper

Ingredient Tip: To clean a leek, slice it in half lengthwise and then soak it in cold water. Agitate the leek in the water so any dirt hiding between the layers comes out. Replace the water and repeat as needed until the leeks are clean.

1. In a large saucepan over medium heat, heat the olive oil. Add the carrots, zucchini, red bell pepper, and leek. Cook for 5 minutes, stirring frequently until the vegetables just begin to soften.

2. Add the chicken stock and bring to a simmer. Stir in the tomato, parsley, thyme, and bay leaf.

3. Add the chicken and simmer for 20 minutes.

4. Season to taste with sea salt and pepper and remove the thyme sprigs and bay leaf. Serve hot.

PER SERVING: Calories: 245, Protein: 29g, Cholesterol: 54mg, Sodium: 1,165mg, Total Carbohydrates: 15g, Fiber: 4g, Total Fat: 8g, Saturated Fat: 2g

CURRIED CHICKEN SOUP

GRAIN-FREE | GLUTEN-FREE | NUT-FREE | SOY-FREE | KID-FRIENDLY | LOW-FODMAP

This mild curry soup is a nice twist on chicken soup that even kids enjoy. Any off-the-shelf curry powder will do. Made with chicken stock and coconut milk, this soup is creamy and delicious.

SERVES 4

Prep time: 10 minutes
Cook time: 20 minutes

1 tablespoon coconut oil
2 tablespoons curry powder
Pinch asafetida
2 boneless skinless chicken breasts,
    cut into thin strips
4 cups Chicken Stock (page 100)
1 (15-ounce) can coconut milk
4 cups roughly chopped
    fresh spinach
Sea salt

Phase 2 Tip: Peas and carrots work really well in this soup. In Phase 2, add ½ cup diced carrots when you add the chicken in step 2, and substitute ½ cup frozen peas for the spinach in step 4.

1. In a large saucepan over medium-high heat, melt the coconut oil. Add the curry powder and asafetida and cook for about 15 seconds, stirring constantly until fragrant.

2. Add the chicken and cook, stirring constantly, until the meat is fully coated and beginning to brown.

3. Add the chicken stock and bring to a boil. Reduce the heat to low and simmer for 15 minutes.

4. Stir in the coconut milk and continue to cook until heated through. Add the spinach and stir until wilted. Season to taste with sea salt and serve.

PER SERVING: Calories: 468, Protein: 30g, Cholesterol: 65mg, Sodium: 984mg, Total Carbohydrates: 10g, Fiber: 4g, Total Fat: 37g, Saturated Fat: 27g

CREAMY PARSNIP SOUP

VEGETARIAN | GRAIN-FREE | GLUTEN-FREE | NUT-FREE | SOY-FREE | KID-FRIENDLY

Parsnips and potatoes form the base of this creamy soup, along with the sweet flavor of leek. Loaded with carotenoids, leeks are a healing food. Because they are so mild, young children tend to love them.

SERVES 4

Prep time: 15 minutes
Cook time: 30 minutes

2 tablespoons butter
2 cups chopped leeks (green
    part only)
1 pound parsnips, peeled and diced
1 medium potato, peeled and diced
2 cups Vegetable Stock (page 99)
2 cups water
1 cup unsweetened coconut milk,
    almond milk, or other
    non-dairy milk
Sea salt
Freshly ground black pepper

Variation Tip: To make this savory soup even better, garnish with a small handful of shredded Cheddar cheese.

1. In a large saucepan over medium heat, melt the butter. Set aside ¼ cup of leeks and add the remainder to the pot. Cook for 5 minutes, stirring constantly until the leeks are tender.

2. Add the parsnips, potato, vegetable stock, and water. Bring to a boil. Reduce the heat to low and simmer for 20 minutes until the parsnips and potatoes are tender.

3. Using an immersion blender, purée the soup. Stir in the coconut milk and season to taste with sea salt and pepper.

4. Divide the soup evenly among 4 bowls and serve garnished with the reserved leeks.

PER SERVING: Calories: 235, Protein: 6g, Cholesterol: 15mg, Sodium: 684mg, Total Carbohydrates: 37g, Fiber: 8g, Total Fat: 8g, Saturated Fat: 5g

TOM KHA GAI

DAIRY-FREE | GLUTEN-FREE | NUT-FREE | SOY-FREE | LOW-FODMAP

This classic Thai soup brings together spicy chiles, astringent lime, sweet coconut cream, and salty fish sauce to make a wonderfully balanced soup. Tofu and shrimp keep this soup light, yet packed with protein. If you like it hot, add more chiles to taste. Be careful not to boil this soup, as this can cause the coconut milk to curdle.

SERVES 4

Prep time: 5 minutes
Cook time: 10 minutes

---

4 cups unsweetened coconut milk

4 stalks lemongrass, cut into
    2-inch pieces

6 (½-inch-thick) slices
    peeled galangal

½ pound medium shrimp, peeled
    and deveined

1 (8-ounce) block firm tofu

1 cup coconut cream

2 red Thai chiles, bruised with
    the handle of a knife

¼ cup fresh lime juice

3 tablespoons fish sauce

Ingredient Tip: Galangal and lemongrass can both be found at most Asian markets. To prepare lemongrass, slice off the root end and remove the outer layer before chopping as directed. Galangal, which looks like ginger, can be easily sliced. If you have extra, slice it and freeze it in a freezer-safe bag or airtight container for about 1 month.

1. In a large pot or wok over medium heat, heat the coconut milk. Add the lemongrass and galangal, and gently simmer for 5 minutes to infuse the milk.

2. Stir in the shrimp and tofu. Cook for 1 to 2 minutes until the shrimp are opaque.

3. Add the coconut cream and stir well.

4. Stir in the chiles and cook for 3 to 4 minutes.

5. Turn off the heat and stir in the lime juice and fish sauce. Serve immediately.

PER SERVING: Calories: 812, Protein: 25g, Cholesterol: 119mg, Sodium: 1,233mg, Total Carbohydrates: 22g, Fiber: 7g, Total Fat: 75g, Saturated Fat: 64g

GREEK SALAD

VEGETARIAN | GLUTEN-FREE | NUT-FREE | SOY-FREE | LOW-FODMAP

There is something about the blend of lemon, feta, and olives in a Greek salad that can't be beat. Perfect for a light lunch or as a side at dinner, this salad is fresh and bursting with flavor. It doesn't take long to prepare, making it a win–win meal.

SERVES 4

Prep time: 10 minutes

1 large head romaine lettuce, finely chopped
1 cup cherry tomatoes, halved
½ cup crumbled feta cheese
⅓ cup Kalamata olives, sliced
3 tablespoons fresh lemon juice
3 tablespoons extra virgin olive oil
½ teaspoon dried oregano
Sea salt
Freshly ground black pepper

Phase 2 Tip: Diced cucumber and red onion plus beautiful heirloom tomatoes are traditional toppings you can add to this salad. To make it even more filling, add 1 or 2 sliced, cooked beets. Beets are loaded with betacyanin, a potent anticarcinogen and the reason behind their striking color.

1. Arrange the lettuce on a large serving plate. Top with the tomatoes, feta, and olives. Set aside.

2. In a small bowl, whisk together the lemon juice, olive oil, and oregano. Season to taste with sea salt and pepper. Drizzle over the salad and serve.

PER SERVING: Calories: 175, Protein: 4g, Cholesterol: 17mg, Sodium: 549mg, Total Carbohydrates: 6g, Fiber: 2g, Total Fat: 16g, Saturated Fat: 5g

HARVEST SALAD WITH POPPY SEED VINAIGRETTE

VEGETARIAN | GRAIN-FREE | GLUTEN-FREE | SOY-FREE | LOW-FODMAP

This salad has a bit of everything: crunch, unexpected sweetness, and a slight tang. Enjoy this bare-bones version while in Phase 1, and be sure to make it with the add-ons in Phase 2 for even more flavor.

SERVES 4

Prep time: 10 minutes

2 heads leaf lettuce, red or green, torn into small pieces

2 small mandarin oranges, peeled and divided into segments

½ cup chopped unsalted walnuts

¼ cup raw unsalted sunflower seeds

4 ounces feta cheese, crumbled

¼ cup extra virgin olive oil

3 tablespoons red wine vinegar

1 tablespoon poppy seeds

Sea salt

Freshly ground black pepper

Phase 2 Tip: Add 1 sliced Granny Smith apple, 2 chopped celery stalks, and ¼ cup of dried unsweetened cranberries.

1. Place the lettuce in a large serving bowl. Add the oranges, walnuts, sunflower seeds, and feta cheese. Toss to combine.

2. In a small bowl, whisk together the olive oil, red wine vinegar, and poppy seeds. Season to taste with sea salt and pepper. Drizzle over the salad, and toss to combine. Divide evenly among 4 plates and serve.

PER SERVING: Calories: 379, Protein: 10g, Cholesterol: 25mg, Sodium: 567mg, Total Carbohydrates: 21g, Fiber: 3g, Total Fat: 31g, Saturated Fat: 7g

COBB SALAD

GLUTEN-FREE | NUT-FREE | SOY-FREE | LOW-FODMAP

An American classic, Cobb salad combines eggs, chicken, avocado, and tomatoes for a hearty and satisfying meal. Even without the traditionally included bacon, this salad does not skimp on flavor. Prep the salad ahead of time so you can simply toss with the dressing come mealtime. If you don't have any cooked chicken, see the Tip below for how to poach a chicken breast.

SERVES 4

Prep time: 20 minutes

---

3 tablespoons white wine vinegar

3 tablespoons extra virgin olive oil

1 tablespoon Dijon mustard

1 teaspoon freshly ground
    black pepper

¼ teaspoon sea salt

8 cups mixed salad greens
    (arugula, leaf lettuce, romaine
    lettuce, mesclun)

1 large boneless skinless chicken
    breast, cooked and
    shredded (see Tip)

2 large hardboiled eggs, chopped

2 tomatoes, diced

1 avocado, pitted, peeled, and diced

1 cucumber, diced

¼ cup crumbled blue cheese

Ingredient Tip: Poaching chicken breasts is easy. Just place a boneless skinless chicken breast in a small saucepan, cover it with lightly salted water, and bring to a boil. Reduce the heat to low and simmer the chicken for 15 minutes, or until cooked through. Remove the chicken from the poaching liquid (discard the liquid) and let it cool.

1. In a small bowl, whisk together the white wine vinegar, olive oil, Dijon mustard, pepper, and sea salt. Set aside.

2. In a large serving bowl, combine the salad greens. Set aside 1 tablespoon of dressing. Pour the remainder over the greens and toss gently to combine.

3. Divide the salad greens evenly among 4 plates. Top each with equal amounts of chicken, egg, tomato, avocado, cucumber, and blue cheese. Drizzle with the reserved tablespoon of dressing and serve.

PER SERVING: Calories: 362, Protein: 18g, Cholesterol: 120mg, Sodium: 337mg, Total Carbohydrates: 14g, Fiber: 6g, Total Fat: 28g, Saturated Fat: 6g

KALE & WALNUT SALAD

VEGETARIAN | GLUTEN-FREE | SOY-FREE | LOW-FODMAP

Kale is a much-touted superfood, and with good reason. This leafy green is packed with vitamins A and C, beta-carotene, and calcium—and it tastes great, too. For salads, choose the darker green lacinato kale (or "dinosaur kale" as it is commonly known), as its texture and flavor is better in uncooked dishes. Make this salad a day in advance and refrigerate so the flavors have a chance to meld.

SERVES 4

Prep time: 10 minutes

1 bunch lacinato kale,
    trimmed, leaves sliced into
    ½-inch-thick strips
3 tablespoons fresh lemon juice
3 tablespoons extra virgin olive oil
⅔ cup grated Parmesan cheese
¼ cup unsalted walnuts, chopped
Sea salt
Freshly ground black pepper

Ingredient Tip: Look for kale that is soft and pliable. If the leaves are dry and papery, the kale is too old.

1. In a large salad bowl, place the kale.

2. In a small bowl, whisk together the lemon juice and olive oil. Pour this over the kale and, using your hands, massage the dressing into the kale for at least 1 minute.

3. Add the Parmesan cheese and walnuts and toss to combine. Season to taste with sea salt and pepper. Serve.

PER SERVING: Calories: 259, Protein: 12g, Cholesterol: 15mg, Sodium: 477mg, Total Carbohydrates: 12g, Fiber: 2g, Total Fat: 20g, Saturated Fat: 5g

KALE & PEAR SALAD

VEGETARIAN | GLUTEN-FREE | NUT-FREE | SOY-FREE

Pear adds a welcome sweetness to this simple raw kale salad. Depending on the season, your pear choices may be limited, but red d'Anjou and Seckel varieties are two favorites for this salad. If you want to prepare the salad in advance, make the entire salad without the pears the day before, and then toss in the pear slices before serving to prevent them from browning.

SERVES 4

Prep time: 15 minutes

---

1 bunch lacinato or curly kale, trimmed, leaves sliced into ½-inch-thick strips

3 tablespoons extra virgin olive oil

2 tablespoons white wine vinegar

1 pear, peeled and thinly sliced

Sea salt

Freshly ground black pepper

2 tablespoons crumbled blue cheese

Ingredient Tip: When cutting kale or any leafy vegetable, remove the stems and stack the leaves in a pile. Roll the leaves up into a small cylinder, and then slice into ½-inch-thick strips.

1. In a large salad bowl, place the kale.

2. In a small bowl, whisk together the olive oil and white wine vinegar. Pour this over the kale and, using your hands, massage the dressing into the kale for at least 1 minute.

3. Add the pear and toss to combine. Season to taste with sea salt and pepper. Garnish with the blue cheese and serve.

PER SERVING: Calories: 174, Protein: 4g, Cholesterol: 3mg, Sodium: 211mg, Total Carbohydrates: 16g, Fiber: 3g, Total Fat: 12g, Saturated Fat: 2g

PARMESAN-QUINOA PATTIES & SPINACH SALAD

VEGETARIAN | GLUTEN-FREE | SOY-FREE | LOW-FODMAP

Savory cheese and quinoa patties on a bed of spinach greens make for a light yet filling meal, perfect for a lunch or simple dinner. While the patties benefit from a 10-minute rest in the refrigerator before cooking, you can make the patties up to 4 hours ahead of time and refrigerate until ready to cook.

SERVES 4

Prep time: 15 minutes
Cook time: 15 minutes

For the patties

¼ cup quick-cooking rolled oats
1¼ cups cooked quinoa
¼ cup grated Parmesan cheese
2 large eggs, beaten
2 tablespoons chopped fresh basil
¼ teaspoon sea salt
1 tablespoon extra virgin olive oil

For the salad

8 cups fresh baby spinach
½ cup halved cherry tomatoes
1 carrot, shredded
2 tablespoons balsamic vinegar
2 tablespoons extra virgin olive oil
Sea salt
Freshly ground black pepper

To make the patties

1. In a blender, process the oats to a fine flour.

2. In a large bowl, combine the oat flour, quinoa, Parmesan cheese, eggs, basil, and sea salt.

3. Using your hands, shape the mixture into 8 small patties, pressing firmly to hold together. Arrange the patties in a single layer on a plate and refrigerate for 10 minutes.

4. In a large skillet over medium heat, heat the olive oil. Cook the patties for 5 to 7 minutes, until the bottom is firm and browned. Using a spatula, flip the patties and cook the other side for about 5 minutes more until well browned. Transfer the patties to a plate lined with paper towel and set aside.

To make the salad

1. In a large bowl, toss together the spinach, tomatoes, and carrot.

2. In a small bowl, whisk together the balsamic vinegar and olive oil. Season to taste with sea salt and pepper. Drizzle the dressing over the spinach and toss to combine.

3. Divide the salad evenly among 4 plates. Top each serving with 2 quinoa patties. Serve immediately.

PER SERVING: Calories: 268, Protein: 11g, Cholesterol: 87mg, Sodium: 509mg, Total Carbohydrates: 22g, Fiber: 4g, Total Fat: 16g, Saturated Fat: 3g

Phase 2 Tip: Add thinly sliced red onion and a handful of dried unsweetened cranberries to the salad for a burst of color and flavor.

BERRYLICIOUS FRUIT SALAD

VEGAN | DAIRY-FREE | GRAIN-FREE | GLUTEN-FREE | NUT-FREE | SOY-FREE |
KID-FRIENDLY | LOW-FODMAP

This salad is packed with vitamin C and antioxidants, making it a great way to start the day, or as a snack or a side dish. If you enjoy fruit for breakfast, but need a little more than just fruit for a long morning, pair this with a side of plain yogurt and a tablespoon of chia seeds for a more filling meal.

SERVES 4

Prep time: 5 minutes

1 cup fresh blueberries

1 cup fresh raspberries

1 cup fresh strawberries, hulled
    and sliced

Juice of 1 orange

10 fresh mint leaves, thinly sliced

Phase 2 Tip: For an even more flavorful salad, add 1 cup each of blackberries and boysenberries. If a little sweetness is desired, add up to 1 tablespoon of pure maple syrup to the orange juice.

1. In a medium bowl, gently combine the blueberries, raspberries, strawberries, and orange juice. Add the mint and gently toss to combine.

2. Serve immediately, or refrigerate for 1 to 2 hours so the fruit can macerate for even more flavor.

PER SERVING: Calories: 71, Protein: 1g, Cholesterol: 0mg, Sodium: 2mg, Total Carbohydrates: 17g, Fiber: 5g, Total Fat: <1g, Saturated Fat: 0g

KIWI, GRAPE & STRAWBERRY SALAD

VEGAN | DAIRY-FREE | GRAIN-FREE | GLUTEN-FREE | NUT-FREE | SOY-FREE | KID-FRIENDLY | LOW-FODMAP

Strawberries are a good source of fiber and vitamins C and A, while grapes are a formidable source of antioxidants. Kiwi, with its distinctive green flesh, is a great source of vitamin C and potassium, and its seeds even contain essential fatty acids. Together, these fruits are an immune-boosting powerhouse. And the bonus—they taste great, too!

SERVES 4

Prep time: 5 minutes

2 kiwi, peeled and sliced

1 cup seedless red grapes, halved

1 cup strawberries, hulled and quartered

1 tablespoon fresh lemon juice

1 tablespoon pure maple syrup

Ingredient Tip: For the best flavor, buy kiwi when they're firm and let sit at room temperature for several days. If you want to buy a large quantity of kiwi, store them in the refrigerator, where they will ripen slowly and stay fresh for weeks.

1. In a small bowl, combine the kiwi, grapes, and strawberries.

2. In another small bowl, whisk together the lemon juice and maple syrup. Pour over the fruit, and stir to combine.

PER SERVING: Calories: 64, Protein: <1g, Cholesterol: 0mg, Sodium: 3mg, Total Carbohydrates: 16g, Fiber: 2g, Total Fat: <1g, Saturated Fat: 0g

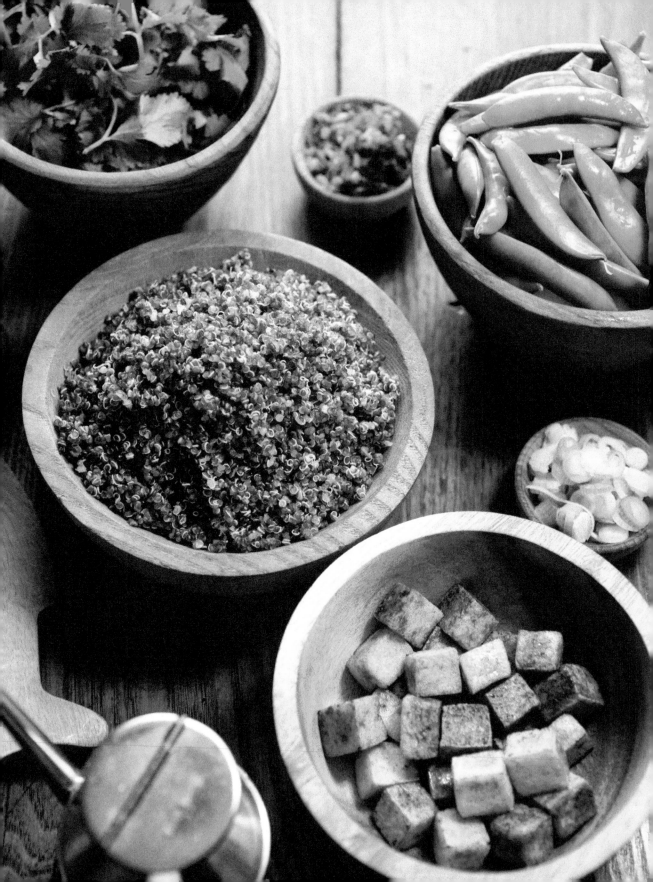

VEGETARIAN & VEGAN SIDES AND MAINS

This chapter is loaded with a variety of sides and main dishes. Pair a simple vegetable side dish with a heartier meat dish from chapter 8, or simply enjoy one of the more substantial vegetarian and vegan sides on its own. Eating a wide variety of naturally colored food livens up your plate and helps you get all the vitamins and minerals you need in your diet.

SAUTÉED GREENS WITH PINE NUTS

VEGAN | DAIRY-FREE | GRAIN-FREE | GLUTEN-FREE | SOY-FREE | LOW-FODMAP

Packed with vitamins and minerals, leafy greens are inexpensive and plentiful throughout the year. This dish is so tasty and takes so little fuss you'll want to serve it at least once a week. The crunchy pine nuts and bitter greens are a delicious pairing.

SERVES 4

Prep time: 10 minutes
Cook time: 10 minutes

¼ cup pine nuts
2 tablespoons extra virgin olive oil
2 bunches mixed greens (kale, collard greens, mustard greens), trimmed and cut into thin strips (see Tip, page 115)
¼ teaspoon red pepper flakes
Sea salt
Red wine vinegar

Phase 2 Tip: In step 3, add ¼ cup of golden raisins along with the pine nuts for a touch of sweetness.

1. In a large dry skillet over medium-high heat, toast the pine nuts for 2 to 3 minutes, shaking the pan frequently until browned. Immediately transfer the toasted pine nuts to a plate.

2. In the same skillet over medium-high heat, heat the olive oil. Add the greens and cook, stirring frequently until they begin to wilt (depending on the type of greens, this will take 1 to 5 minutes). Cover the pan, reduce the heat to low, and cook for 2 to 5 minutes more until the greens are tender.

3. Stir in the toasted pine nuts and red pepper flakes. Add a pinch of sea salt and a splash of red wine vinegar. Toss to combine and cook until any liquid in the pan evaporates. Serve immediately.

PER SERVING: Calories: 131, Protein: 3g, Cholesterol: 0mg, Sodium: 165mg, Total Carbohydrates: 3g, Fiber: 2g, Total Fat: 13g, Saturated Fat: 2g

SAUTÉED SWISS CHARD WITH BALSAMIC VINEGAR

VEGAN | DAIRY-FREE | GRAIN-FREE | GLUTEN-FREE | NUT-FREE | SOY-FREE | LOW-FODMAP

Swiss chard is a quick-cooking green with a distinct buttery taste. Unlike other leafy greens whose stalks are usually discarded, the stalks of Swiss chard are arguably the best part of the green. Because they take a bit longer to cook, the stalks are diced and sautéed ahead of the greens.

SERVES 4

Prep time: 5 minutes
Cook time: 10 minutes

---

2 bunches Swiss chard
2 tablespoons extra virgin olive oil
Pinch asafetida
Sea salt
2 tablespoons balsamic vinegar

Ingredient Tip: There are several varieties of Swiss chard: white, red, and rainbow. Color aside, they all taste quite similar and can be used interchangeably.

1. Separate the greens from the stalks: lay each piece of chard on a cutting board, fold the leaf in half along the stalk, and cut the leaf away from the stalk with a sharp knife, sorting the stalks and greens into separate piles. Cut the greens into 1-inch shreds. Dice the stalks.

2. In a medium skillet over medium-high heat, heat the olive oil. Add the asafetida and a pinch of sea salt and cook for about 45 seconds, stirring constantly until fragrant.

3. Add the diced chard stalks and cook for 3 to 5 minutes, stirring constantly until they begin to soften. Add the greens and cook, stirring occasionally just until they begin to wilt. Cover and reduce the heat to low. Cook for 2 to 3 minutes more until the stalks and greens are tender.

4. Stir in the balsamic vinegar to incorporate. Cook for 1 to 2 minutes until any liquid in the pan evaporates. Serve.

PER SERVING: Calories: 72, Protein: 1g, Cholesterol: 0mg, Sodium: 233mg, Total Carbohydrates: 2g, Fiber: 1g, Total Fat: 7g, Saturated Fat: 1g

ROASTED BUTTERNUT SQUASH

VEGAN | DAIRY-FREE | GRAIN-FREE | GLUTEN-FREE | NUT-FREE | SOY-FREE |
KID-FRIENDLY | LOW-FODMAP

Butternut squash is a variety of winter squash, which means it is in season in late summer and fall. It has a hard skin that makes it perfect for overwinter storage—it will keep in a dark, cool place for up to six months and is available at the grocery store year-round. Full of phytonutrients and antioxidants, it has "superfood" status, yet it is an often-overlooked vegetable, in large part because many people aren't sure how to prepare it. Roasting it, as in this recipe, results in a sweet, warming, delicious side dish.

SERVES 4

Prep time: 10 minutes
Cook time: 30 minutes

2 tablespoons extra virgin olive oil
1 tablespoon pure maple syrup
1 teaspoon sea salt
1 teaspoon freshly ground black
    pepper
1 large butternut squash, halved,
    seeded, peeled, and cubed

Ingredient Tip: To remove the skin easily from butternut squash, cut the squash in half and scoop out the seeds. Place the two halves cut-side down on a microwave-safe dish with a couple tablespoons of water on the dish. Microwave for 2 minutes on high. When the squash is cool enough to handle, you'll be able to remove the softened skin using a vegetable peeler. You can also find bags of peeled and cubed squash at the supermarket.

1. Preheat the oven to 400°F.

2. Line a baking sheet with parchment paper.

3. In a large bowl, whisk together the olive oil, maple syrup, sea salt, and pepper. Add the squash and toss until well coated. Arrange the squash on the prepared baking sheet in a single layer.

4. Bake in the preheated oven for 30 minutes, turning the squash halfway through. Serve warm.

PER SERVING: Calories: 122, Protein: 1g, Cholesterol: 0mg, Sodium: 473mg, Total Carbohydrates: 16g, Fiber: 2g, Total Fat: 7g, Saturated Fat: 1g

ROASTED POTATOES & SWEET POTATOES

VEGAN | DAIRY-FREE | GRAIN-FREE | GLUTEN-FREE | NUT-FREE | SOY-FREE | KID-FRIENDLY

Choose an orange-fleshed variety of sweet potato to benefit from its high levels of beta-carotene and for a lovely presentation alongside the new potatoes. Sweet potatoes are nutrient dense and can help stabilize blood sugar levels, making them a great addition to your table, especially when serving other starchy vegetables, such as white potatoes.

SERVES 6

Prep time: 10 minutes
Cook time: 35 minutes

---

1 pound new potatoes, cut into
    ¾-inch cubes
1 pound sweet potatoes, cut into
    ¾-inch cubes
1 tablespoon extra virgin olive oil
Sea salt
Freshly ground black pepper
1 tablespoon fresh flat-leaf
    Italian parsley, chopped

Time-Saving Tip: Use any leftover potatoes and sweet potatoes in the Quinoa & Roasted Vegetable Bowl (page 136) as a substitute for the butternut squash.

1. Preheat the oven to 450°F.

2. Line a baking sheet with parchment paper.

3. In a large bowl, toss together the new potatoes, sweet potatoes, and olive oil. Season to taste with sea salt and pepper.

4. Spread the potatoes on the prepared sheet and roast for 20 minutes. Use a spatula to loosen and flip the potatoes. Rotate the baking sheet and continue to cook for 15 minutes more until the potatoes are golden brown. Sprinkle with parsley to garnish and serve immediately.

PER SERVING: Calories: 162, Protein: 3g, Cholesterol: 0mg, Sodium: 168mg, Total Carbohydrates: 33g, Fiber: 4g, Total Fat: 3g, Saturated Fat: 0g

SPICED KABOCHA SQUASH

VEGAN | DAIRY-FREE | GRAIN-FREE | NUT-FREE | LOW-FODMAP

Kabocha, a Japanese winter squash, is widely available throughout the United States and is a colorful addition to any meal. Unlike many other types of winter squash, the skin of kabocha is completely edible and lends a wonderful crisp texture to this dish. Slightly spicy, this warming side dish is packed with beta-carotene and pairs well with pork and chicken.

SERVES 4

Prep time: 10 minutes
Cook time: 25 minutes

- ½ teaspoon ground cumin
- ¼ teaspoon cayenne pepper
- ¼ teaspoon ground cinnamon
- ¼ teaspoon ground nutmeg
- ¼ teaspoon sea salt
- ½ medium kabocha squash, halved, seeded, and cut into ½-inch cubes
- 2 tablespoons pure maple syrup
- 1 tablespoon soy sauce
- 2 teaspoons toasted sesame oil

Ingredient Tips: Kabocha squash are often sold pre-cut in half, which saves some time as this is one tough squash. To prepare a squash yourself, carefully insert the tip of a sharp knife into the stem and then push the knife straight down, holding the squash steady to prevent it from slipping. Repeat directly across from your first incision. Then, using your hands, pull the squash apart and scoop out the seeds with a large spoon. If you don't have any toasted sesame oil on hand, you can substitute extra virgin olive oil.

1. Preheat the oven to 400°F.

2. Line a baking sheet with parchment paper.

3. In a large bowl, combine the cumin, cayenne pepper, cinnamon, nutmeg, and sea salt. Add the squash and toss until well coated. Add the maple syrup and soy sauce, and toss again until well coated. Arrange the squash in a single layer on the prepared baking sheet. Drizzle lightly with the sesame oil.

4. Bake in the preheated oven for 10 minutes. Using a spatula, turn the squash pieces over, and continue to bake for 15 minutes more until lightly browned and beginning to crisp around the edges. Serve.

PER SERVING: Calories: 98, Protein: 1g, Cholesterol: 0mg, Sodium: 348mg, Total Carbohydrates: 20g, Fiber: 2g, Total Fat: 3g, Saturated Fat: 0g

CURRIED SQUASH BOWLS

VEGAN | DAIRY-FREE | GRAIN-FREE | GLUTEN-FREE | NUT-FREE | SOY-FREE | LOW-FODMAP

Acorn squash—a squat, compact green variety of squash available year-round—makes the perfect single-serving vegetable, especially when all you need to do is sprinkle it with curry powder and maple syrup. So easy, yet so good.

SERVES 4

Prep time: 5 minutes
Cook time: 20 to 30 minutes

---

4 small acorn squash
2 teaspoons curry powder
½ teaspoon sea salt
2 tablespoons extra virgin olive oil
1 tablespoon pure maple syrup
Freshly ground black pepper

Ingredient Tip: Don't toss those squash seeds! Like pumpkin seeds, you can roast them for a delicious and nutritious treat. Rinse the pulp from the seeds under cold running water and dry well. Place the seeds in a bowl and toss with 1 teaspoon of olive oil and a dash of sea salt. Spread over a baking sheet and roast along with the squash for 15 to 20 minutes at 425°F, stirring occasionally.

1. Preheat the oven to 425°F.

2. Using a sharp knife, cut the stem ends from the squash to create "bowls." Carefully scoop out the seeds using a sturdy spoon (reserve the seeds; see Tip). Place the squash cut-side up on a baking sheet. Sprinkle the inside of each squash with the curry powder and sea salt.

3. In a small bowl, whisk together the olive oil and maple syrup. Drizzle evenly over each squash.

4. Roast in the preheated oven for 20 to 30 minutes, stirring once or twice, until the squash is tender and can be easily pierced with a fork. Season to taste with pepper and serve.

PER SERVING: Calories: 249, Protein: 4g, Cholesterol: 0mg, Sodium: 248mg, Total Carbohydrates: 49g, Fiber: 7g, Total Fat: 8g, Saturated Fat: 1g

RUTABAGA FRIES

VEGAN | DAIRY-FREE | GRAIN-FREE | GLUTEN-FREE | NUT-FREE |
SOY-FREE | KID-FRIENDLY | LOW-FODMAP

Another underused vegetable in the kitchen, rutabaga (a cross between a turnip and a cabbage) is sweet and earthy. Because this bulbous vegetable retains a bit of firmness when "oven fried," it's a perfect stand-in for potatoes during Phase 1.

SERVES 4

Prep time: 5 minutes
Cook time: 30 minutes

---

1 large rutabaga
1 tablespoon extra virgin olive oil
¼ teaspoon sea salt
¼ teaspoon freshly ground
    black pepper

Variation Tip: For a little extra flavor, add 2 tablespoons of finely chopped fresh rosemary along with the olive oil and bake as directed.

1. Preheat the oven to 400°F.

2. Line a baking sheet with parchment paper.

3. Using a paring knife, peel the rutabaga. Cut into ½-inch rounds and then cut each round into ½-inch-thick strips.

4. In a large bowl, combine the rutabaga strips, olive oil, sea salt, and pepper, and toss until well coated. Arrange the rutabaga strips in a single layer on the prepared baking sheet.

5. Bake in the preheated oven for 30 minutes, checking the fries every 10 minutes and turning them at least once. When they can be easily pierced with a fork, the fries are ready. Serve warm.

PER SERVING: Calories: 100, Protein: 2g, Cholesterol: 0mg, Sodium: 156mg, Total Carbohydrates: 16g, Fiber: 5g, Total Fat: 4g, Saturated Fat: <1g

MASHED CELERIAC

VEGETARIAN | GRAIN-FREE | GLUTEN-FREE | SOY-FREE | KID-FRIENDLY | LOW-FODMAP

Celeriac is related to common celery, but grown only for its lumpy, brownish root. You can find it in the vegetable section of any well-stocked supermarket or health food store. Cooked and mashed, it has an earthy flavor that is a cross between turnips, potatoes, and celery. Celeriac can also be eaten raw and is especially delicious when grated and dressed with a vinaigrette.

SERVES 4

Prep time: 5 minutes
Cook time: 25 minutes

2 large celeriac
1 tablespoon extra virgin olive oil
Pinch asafetida
1 teaspoon sea salt
¼ teaspoon freshly ground
    black pepper
5 cups water
1 tablespoon butter
¼ cup unsweetened almond milk
    or coconut milk

Phase 2 Tip: Add 1 or 2 cooked potatoes cooked to the pan in step 3. Combining potatoes and celeriac in a mash is a great way to introduce celeriac to picky eaters without a fuss.

Variation Tip: You can make mashed rutabaga using this recipe with great results. Simply substitute 1 large rutabaga for the celeriac in step 1.

1. Using a sharp knife, trim off the top and bottom ends of the celeriac. Rinse under cool running water to remove any dirt. Using a paring knife, peel and then rinse again to remove any remaining dirt. Cut into ½-inch rounds and then into ½-inch cubes.

2. In a large saucepan over medium-high heat, heat the olive oil. Add the asafetida, sea salt, and pepper and cook for about 45 seconds, stirring constantly until fragrant.

3. Add the celeriac and cook for 5 minutes until it begins to soften. Add the water, increase the heat to high, and bring to a boil. Reduce the heat to low and simmer for 20 minutes or until fork tender.

4. Using a colander, drain the celeriac and return it to the saucepan. Using a potato masher, mash until smooth.

5. Stir in the butter and almond milk. Taste and adjust the seasoning, if desired. Serve.

PER SERVING: Calories: 156, Protein: 3g, Cholesterol: 8mg, Sodium: 656mg, Total Carbohydrates: 15g, Fiber: 3g, Total Fat: 10g, Saturated Fat: 6g

ROASTED ASPARAGUS

VEGETARIAN | GRAIN-FREE | GLUTEN-FREE | NUT-FREE | SOY-FREE

Asparagus is packed with bioflavonoids known for their immune-strengthening, antioxidant, and anticarcinogenic properties. In fact, asparagus is one of the top five vegetable sources of glutathione, a powerful bioflavonoid that plays a role in regulating other antioxidants, such as vitamins A and E. Surprisingly, for a vegetable, it is also a formidable source of protein. This simple preparation lets asparagus's unique flavor shine.

SERVES 4

Prep time: 5 minutes
Cook time: 20 minutes

---

1 pound asparagus, tough ends
   removed
1 tablespoon extra virgin olive oil
Sea salt
Freshly ground black pepper
Juice of ½ lemon
2 tablespoons grated
   Parmesan cheese

Variation Tip: Add a small handful of pine nuts or slivered almonds to the top of the cooked asparagus for additional flavor and a bit of crunch.

1. Preheat the oven to 400°F.

2. Line a large baking sheet with parchment paper.

3. Arrange the asparagus in a single layer on the prepared baking sheet and drizzle with the olive oil. Season to taste with sea salt and pepper. Give the tray several good shakes to coat the asparagus in the oil.

4. Roast in the preheated oven for 15 to 20 minutes until crisp tender.

5. Remove the pan from the oven. Squeeze lemon juice over the asparagus. Sprinkle with Parmesan cheese and serve.

PER SERVING: Calories: 66, Protein: 4g, Cholesterol: 3mg, Sodium: 271mg, Total Carbohydrates: 5g, Fiber: 2g, Total Fat: 5g, Saturated Fat: 1g

ROASTED JERUSALEM ARTICHOKES

VEGAN | DAIRY-FREE | GRAIN-FREE | GLUTEN-FREE | NUT-FREE | SOY-FREE

Also called sunchokes, Jerusalem artichokes are nothing like the more commonly recognizable globe artichokes. These unusual tubers look similar to ginger, with a thin brown knobby skin that can be left intact. A great source of the prebiotic inulin, sunchokes are a tasty addition to your menu plan.

SERVES 4

Prep time: 5 minutes
Cook time: 45 minutes

1 pound Jerusalem artichokes, halved
2 tablespoons extra virgin olive oil
Sea salt
Freshly ground black pepper
1 sprig fresh rosemary, leaves minced

Ingredient Tip: Jerusalem artichokes can be difficult for some people to digest due to their high level of inulin, which can cause gastric pain. If this is your first time trying Jerusalem artichokes, start with just one or two pieces and see how your body handles them.

1. Preheat the oven to 425°F.

2. Line a baking sheet with parchment paper.

3. Place the artichokes in a large bowl. Add the olive oil and season to taste with sea salt and pepper. Toss until well coated.

4. Arrange the coated artichokes in a single layer on the prepared baking sheet. Sprinkle with the rosemary.

5. Bake in the preheated oven for 45 minutes, until tender and easily pierced with a fork, turning once half way though the cooking time. Serve warm.

PER SERVING: Calories: 113, Protein: 4g, Cholesterol: 0mg, Sodium: 224mg, Total Carbohydrates: 12g, Fiber: 6g, Total Fat: 7g, Saturated Fat: 1g

CAULIFLOWER RICE

VEGAN | DAIRY-FREE | GLUTEN-FREE | NUT-FREE | SOY-FREE | KID-FRIENDLY

A paleo-friendly play on rice, this cauliflower dish makes a great base for stews and curries. Cauliflower is also a good source of vitamins C, K, and B$_6$, folate, pantothenic acid, potassium, and manganese. Pack leftovers for lunch the next day and eat it warm or cold.

SERVES 4

Prep time: 15 minutes
Cook time: 15 minutes

1 small head cauliflower,
   cut into florets
1 teaspoon extra virgin olive oil
1 garlic clove, chopped
½ teaspoon sea salt
Pinch freshly ground black pepper
2 teaspoons fresh lemon juice

Cooking Tip: If you don't have a food processor, you can grate the cauliflower using a box grater to achieve the same rice-like texture.

1. In a food processor fitted with the metal blade, process the cauliflower florets until they resemble the texture of rice.

2. In a large skillet over medium heat, combine the olive oil and garlic and sauté for 1 to 2 minutes until the garlic is slightly browned.

3. Add the cauliflower "rice," sea salt, and pepper. Cook for about 10 minutes, stirring constantly until the cauliflower begins to brown.

4. Remove the pan from the heat and stir in the lemon juice. Serve.

PER SERVING: Calories: 28, Protein: 1g, Cholesterol: 0mg, Sodium: 255mg, Total Carbohydrates: 4g, Fiber: 2g, Total Fat: 1g, Saturated Fat: 0g

CAULIFLOWER RICE PILAF

VEGAN | DAIRY-FREE | GRAIN-FREE | GLUTEN-FREE | SOY-FREE | KID-FRIENDLY

This satisfying faux-rice pilaf tastes as good as it looks and makes an impressive side dish.

SERVES 4

Prep time: 10 minutes
Cook time: 10 minutes

1 large head cauliflower,
   cut into florets
2 tablespoons extra virgin olive oil
Pinch asafetida
½ cup Vegetable Stock (page 99)
Sea salt
½ cup golden raisins
½ cup slivered almonds
¼ cup chopped fresh flat-leaf
   Italian parsley

Variation Tip: For added color, substitute dried unsweetened cranberries for the raisins. If desired, you can also substitute hazelnuts or walnuts for the almonds.

1. In a food processor fitted with the metal blade, process the cauliflower florets until they resemble the texture of rice (you can also grate it on the large holes of a box grater). Set aside.

2. In a medium skillet over medium-high heat, heat the olive oil. Add the asafetida and cook for about 45 seconds, stirring constantly until fragrant.

3. Add the cauliflower "rice" and cook for 2 to 3 minutes, stirring constantly until the cauliflower softens slightly.

4. Stir in the vegetable stock and season to taste. Reduce the heat to low, cover, and cook for 5 minutes more until the cauliflower is tender.

5. Remove from the heat and gently fold in the raisins, almonds, and parsley. Taste and adjust the seasonings, if desired. Serve.

PER SERVING: Calories: 206, Protein: 5g, Cholesterol: 0mg, Sodium: 237mg, Total Carbohydrates: 21g, Fiber: 4g, Total Fat: 13g, Saturated Fat: 2g

TOFU & QUINOA BOWL WITH SNAP PEAS

VEGAN | DAIRY-FREE | GRAIN-FREE | GLUTEN-FREE | NUT-FREE | SOY-FREE

Lightly pan-fried tofu, fresh sugar snap peas, lemony cilantro, and a lime vinaigrette round out this filling quinoa bowl. Because this recipe is for Phase 2, you can use part of the scallion whites for added bite, if desired.

SERVES 4

Prep time: 10 minutes
Cook time: 25 minutes

1 cup quinoa, rinsed and drained
2 cups Vegetable Stock (page 99)
    or water
1 tablespoon plus 2 teaspoons extra
    virgin olive oil, divided
8 ounces firm tofu, cut into
    1-inch squares
1 cup sugar snap peas, trimmed
¼ cup chopped fresh cilantro leaves
Juice of 2 limes
Sea salt
Freshly ground black pepper
2 tablespoons chopped scallions
    (green and white parts, as
    desired, for garnish)

Variation Tip: Use premarinated tofu, if desired: Tamari, ginger, and garlic tofu all work well in this recipe.

1. In a small saucepan, combine the quinoa and vegetable stock and bring to a boil. Cover, reduce the heat to low, and simmer for about 15 minutes until the liquid is completely absorbed. Using a fork, fluff the cooked quinoa. Set aside until cooled to room temperature.

2. In a skillet over medium-high heat, heat 1 tablespoon of olive oil. Using a paper towel or a clean kitchen towel, pat the tofu dry. Cook the tofu for about 4 minutes per side until golden brown all over. Transfer to a plate lined with paper towel.

3. In a large bowl, combine the cooked quinoa, cooked tofu, sugar snap peas, and cilantro. Drizzle with the remaining 2 teaspoons of olive oil and the lime juice and toss to combine. Season to taste with sea salt and pepper. Serve garnished with the scallions.

PER SERVING: Calories: 285, Protein: 14g, Cholesterol: 0mg, Sodium: 511mg, Total Carbohydrates: 34g, Fiber: 5g, Total Fat: 12g, Saturated Fat: 2g

QUINOA & ROASTED VEGETABLE BOWL

VEGETARIAN | GLUTEN-FREE | SOY-FREE | LOW-FODMAP

Roasted vegetables take the main stage in this quinoa bowl. Loaded with carrots, fennel, butternut squash, and Brussels sprouts, this makes a filling and warming lunch or dinner.

SERVES 4

Prep time: 10 minutes
Cook time: 35 minutes

———

2 carrots, peeled and cut into
    1-inch rounds
1 small fennel bulb, sliced into
    thin wedges
¾ pound Brussels sprouts
½ butternut squash, halved, seeded,
    peeled and cut into 1-inch cubes
4 tablespoons extra virgin
    olive oil, divided
1 teaspoon sea salt, divided
½ teaspoon freshly ground black
    pepper, divided
½ teaspoon red pepper flakes
¾ cup quinoa, rinsed and drained
1½ cups Vegetable Stock (page 99)
2 cups fresh baby spinach
2 tablespoons red wine vinegar
¼ cup unsalted walnuts, broken into
    small pieces
¼ cup crumbled feta cheese

1. Preheat the oven to 400°F.

2. In a large bowl, combine the carrots, fennel, Brussels sprouts, and squash. Sprinkle with 2 tablespoons of olive oil, ½ teaspoon of sea salt, ¼ teaspoon of black pepper, and the red pepper flakes. Arrange the vegetables in a single layer on a large baking sheet and bake in the preheated oven for 20 minutes.

3. Increase the oven temperature to 425°F and bake for 10 to 15 minutes more until the vegetables are browned and tender.

4. Meanwhile, in a small pot, combine the quinoa and vegetable stock and bring to a boil. Cover, reduce the heat to low, and simmer for 15 minutes, or until the liquid is completely absorbed. Using a fork, fluff the cooked quinoa.

5. Add the spinach and stir to combine. Cover and let steam for about 2 minutes until the spinach is wilted. Uncover and set aside until cooled to room temperature.

6. Into the cooled quinoa, stir the remaining
2 tablespoons of olive oil, ½ teaspoon of sea salt,
¼ teaspoon of black pepper, and the red wine vinegar.

7. To serve, divide the quinoa among 4 serving bowls
and top with the roasted vegetables, walnuts, and
feta cheese.

PER SERVING: Calories: 404, Protein: 14g, Cholesterol: 6mg,
Sodium: 914mg, Total Carbohydrates: 41g, Fiber: 9g,
Total Fat: 23g, Saturated Fat: 4g

*Time-Saving Tip: Cooked quinoa
will keep for 3 to 4 days in an airtight
container in the refrigerator, so you
may want to double the amount you
cook to have some on hand for later
in the week.*

ZUCCHINI RICE BOATS

VEGETARIAN | GLUTEN-FREE | NUT-FREE | SOY-FREE

These zucchini boats are a great way to turn leftover cooked rice into an attractive side dish. Small zucchini are convenient for serving, but you can also make this dish with one larger zucchini (just increase the roasting time slightly). The filling also pairs well with other kinds of cooked squash, such as butternut.

SERVES 4

Prep time: 10 minutes
Cook time: 30 minutes

---

4 small zucchini, ends removed
   and halved lengthwise
1 teaspoon extra virgin olive oil
3 garlic cloves, chopped
4 cups roughly chopped fresh
   spinach leaves
½ teaspoon sea salt
3 cups cooked long-grain white rice
½ cup whipping (35 percent) cream
½ cup cooked black beans
½ cup dehydrated sun-dried
   tomatoes, diced
¼ cup grated Parmesan cheese

Cooking Tip: For added fiber, use long-grain brown rice or a mixture of white and brown rice.

1. Preheat the oven to 350°F.

2. Using a spoon, hollow out a 1-inch "trench" down the center of each zucchini half. Arrange the zucchini cut-side up on a baking sheet.

3. Bake in the preheated oven for 15 minutes or until the zucchini are tender. Remove from the oven.

4. In a skillet over medium-low heat, heat the olive oil. Add the garlic and sauté for 2 to 3 minutes until just starting to brown.

5. Add the spinach and sauté until it wilts.

6. Add the sea salt, rice, whipping cream, black beans, and sun-dried tomatoes, and stir well. Cook until everything is heated through.

7. Remove the pan from the heat. Using a spoon, fill each zucchini half with an equal amount of the rice mixture, packing it down tightly. Sprinkle with the Parmesan cheese and place on the baking sheet.

8. Set the oven to broil.

9. Return the sheet to the oven and broil for 2 to 3 minutes, or until the cheese begins to brown. Serve.

PER SERVING: Calories: 458, Protein: 16g, Cholesterol: 22mg, Sodium: 354mg, Total Carbohydrates: 81g, Fiber: 8g, Total Fat: 9g, Saturated Fat: 4g

TURMERIC-SPICED QUINOA SALAD

VEGAN | DAIRY-FREE | GLUTEN-FREE | NUT-FREE | SOY-FREE

Turmeric is a powerful anti-inflammatory, and just about everyone should be eating more of this brightly colored spice. Here, turmeric is paired with cilantro, parsley, quinoa, and avocado for a delightfully quick and simple meal.

SERVES 4

Prep time: 5 minutes
Cook time: 20 minutes

1½ cups quinoa, rinsed and drained
3 cups Vegetable Stock (page 99)
    or water
2 teaspoons coconut oil
Pinch asafetida
½ cup chopped fresh flat-leaf Italian
    parsley leaves
1 teaspoon sea salt
1 teaspoon ground cumin
1 teaspoon ground turmeric
½ teaspoon freshly crushed
    black pepper
1 avocado, pitted, peeled,
    and diced, divided
1 cup chopped fresh cilantro
    leaves, divided

Variation Tip: If desired, serve the cooked quinoa salad with lettuce or kale leaves for a simple rollup that is perfect finger food.

1. In a small pot over medium-high heat, combine the quinoa and vegetable stock and bring to a boil. Cover, reduce the heat to low, and simmer for 15 minutes until the liquid is completely absorbed. Using a fork, fluff the cooked quinoa.

2. In a skillet over medium-high heat, heat the coconut oil. Add the asafetida and cook for about 45 seconds, stirring constantly until fragrant.

3. Add the parsley and sauté for about 1 minute until fragrant.

4. Add the sea salt, cumin, turmeric, and pepper. Cook for about 30 seconds, stirring quickly to prevent scorching. Add the cooked quinoa and stir well.

5. To serve, divide the quinoa mixture among 4 serving bowls and top with equal portions of avocado and cilantro.

PER SERVING: Calories: 394, Protein: 14g, Cholesterol: 0mg, Sodium: 1,054mg, Total Carbohydrates: 47g, Fiber: 8g, Total Fat: 17g, Saturated Fat: 5g

MEDITERRANEAN SORGHUM BOWL

VEGETARIAN | GLUTEN-FREE | NUT-FREE | SOY-FREE | LOW-FODMAP

A staple grain in Africa and Asian, sorghum is a popular cereal crop that has been cultivated for over 5,000 years. This filling, gluten-free bowl is bright and flavorful, loaded with feta cheese, cucumbers, tomatoes, and olives and drizzled with a lemon.

SERVES 4

Prep time: 15 minutes
Cook time: 45 minutes

3½ cups water

1¼ cups sorghum grains, rinsed
    and drained

Zest of 2 lemons

Juice of 2 lemons

2 tablespoons extra virgin olive oil

1 teaspoon sea salt

½ teaspoon freshly ground
    black pepper

2 cups cherry tomatoes,
    halved, divided

1 large cucumber, cut into ½-inch
    cubes, divided

1 cup pitted Kalamata olives,
    halved, divided

1 cup crumbled feta cheese, divided

2 cups fresh baby spinach, divided

Time-Saving Tip: Sorghum takes longer to cook than other grains, so it is helpful to cook a large batch in a slow cooker to use later. Add 3 cups of water for every 1 cup of sorghum, and cook for 4 hours on high. Cool and refrigerate leftovers in an airtight container for up to 3 days, or freeze for 1 month.

1. In a saucepan, combine the water and sorghum and bring to a boil. Reduce the heat to low, cover, and simmer for 45 minutes until the liquid is completely absorbed and the sorghum is tender.

2. In a small bowl, whisk together the lemon zest, lemon juice, olive oil, sea salt, and pepper.

3. Divide the cooked sorghum among 4 serving bowls. Top with equal amounts of tomatoes, cucumbers, olives, feta cheese, and spinach. Drizzle with the lemon vinaigrette, and serve.

PER SERVING: Calories: 504, Protein: 6g, Cholesterol: 25mg, Sodium: 1,103mg, Total Carbohydrates: 87g, Fiber: 3g, Total Fat: 17g, Saturated Fat: 6g

VEGETABLE MILLET BOWL WITH TAHINI DRESSING

VEGAN | DAIRY-FREE | GLUTEN-FREE | NUT-FREE | SOY-FREE

Millet is a member of the grass family and has been cultivated for thousands of years. It is a cereal grain, and boasts an impressive amino acid content, as well as a high iron content. It is super easy to digest and makes a great bed for a whole host of toppings. In this bowl, it is topped with a savory tahini dressing and loaded with fresh vegetables.

SERVES 4

Prep time: 10 minutes
Cook time: 20 minutes

For the tahini dressing

1 cup tahini
⅓ cup water
¼ cup fresh lemon juice
Sea salt

For the bowl

2 cups water
1 cup millet, rinsed and drained
2 tablespoons toasted sesame oil
2 tablespoons apple cider vinegar
2 carrots, shredded, divided
1 cucumber, diced, divided
2 cups baby kale, divided
**1 avocado, pitted, peeled, and
    diced, divided**

Phase 2 Tip: For added protein, divide 1 (15-ounce) can of rinsed and drained black beans or garbanzo beans (chickpeas) among the bowls.

To make the tahini dressing

In a small bowl, whisk together the tahini, water, and lemon juice. Season to taste with sea salt. If needed, add a little more water to make a thinner dressing. Set aside.

To make the bowl

1. In a small saucepan, combine the water and millet and bring to a boil. Reduce the heat to low, cover, and simmer for 20 minutes until the liquid is completely absorbed. Using a fork, fluff the cooked millet. Stir in the sesame oil and apple cider vinegar.

2. Divide the cooked millet among 4 serving bowls. Top each bowl with an equal amount of carrots, cucumbers, kale, and avocado. Drizzle with the tahini dressing and serve.

PER SERVING: Calories: 754, Protein: 19g, Cholesterol: 0mg, Sodium: 232mg, Total Carbohydrates: 63g, Fiber: 15g, Total Fat: 51g, Saturated Fat: 8g

BUCKWHEAT TABBOULEH WITH AVOCADO & CHICKPEAS

VEGAN | DAIRY-FREE | GLUTEN-FREE | NUT-FREE | SOY-FREE

Buckwheat groats are the hulled seeds of the buckwheat plant and hold up to cooking the same way a wheat or cereal grain does. Buckwheat boasts the longest transit time in the gut, leaving you feeling full for longer. It also has a remarkably high proportion of all the essential amino acids, making it a good source of protein in your diet.

SERVES 4

Prep time: 10 minutes
Cook time: 10 to 15 minutes

1½ cups Vegetable Stock (page 99) or water

1 cup buckwheat groats

6 scallions (green and white parts, as desired), thinly sliced

¼ cup chopped fresh flat-leaf Italian parsley leaves

2 tablespoons chopped fresh cilantro

Juice of 2 lemons

1 tablespoon extra virgin olive oil

Sea salt

Freshly ground black pepper

8 radishes, sliced, divided

1 (15-ounce) can garbanzo beans, divided

1 avocado, pitted, peeled, and thinly sliced, divided

Variation Tip: Turn this into a wrap! Serve the tabbouleh with 3 to 4 large lettuce leaves per person.

1. In a saucepan over medium-high heat, combine the vegetable stock and buckwheat groats and bring to a boil. Cook, uncovered, for 8 to 10 minutes until the water is nearly absorbed. Reduce the heat to low, cover the pan, and continue to cook for 2 to 3 minutes more until all the water is absorbed. Using a fork, fluff the cooked buckwheat. Set aside to cool.

2. In a large bowl, combine the cooled buckwheat, scallions, parsley, and cilantro. Set aside.

3. In a small bowl, whisk together the lemon juice and olive oil. Season to taste with sea salt and pepper. Pour the dressing over the buckwheat mixture and stir gently to combine.

4. Divide the salad among 4 serving bowls. Top each serving with radish slices, ¼ cup of garbanzo beans, and one-fourth of the avocado. Serve.

PER SERVING: Calories: 648, Protein: 28g, Cholesterol: 0mg, Sodium: 565mg, Total Carbohydrates: 93g, Fiber: 26g, Total Fat: 21g, Saturated Fat: 4g

BOK CHOY & MACADAMIA STIR-FRY

VEGAN | DAIRY-FREE | LOW-FODMAP

Macadamia nuts are nutritional powerhouses, loaded with more monounsaturated fat than any other nut. Paired with bok choy and served over rice, their sweet, buttery flavor elevates this easy and nutritious stir-fry.

SERVES 4

Prep time: 5 minutes
Cook time: 10 minutes

1 tablespoon extra virgin olive oil
1 large head bok choy, chopped into
   fine strips
1-inch piece peeled fresh
   ginger, minced
Pinch asafetida
½ teaspoon sea salt
½ teaspoon freshly cracked
   black pepper
2 tablespoons soy sauce
1 ounce unsalted macadamia nuts

Phase 2 Tip: Substitute 2 pounds of asparagus for the bok choy or substitute a large head of broccoli for the bok choy and toasted sesame seeds for the macadamia nuts. Serve the stir fry over rice alongside some Korean Kimchi (page 245).

1. In a large skillet or wok over medium-high heat, heat the olive oil. Add the bok choy, ginger, and asafetida. Cook for 5 to 6 minutes, stirring frequently until the bok choy greens wilt and the stems soften slightly. Season with the sea salt and pepper.

2. Add the soy sauce and macadamia nuts. Cook, for 2 to 3 minutes more, stirring constantly until the nuts are coated with sauce and everything is heated through. Serve.

PER SERVING: Calories: 95, Protein: 2g, Cholesterol: 0mg, Sodium: 731mg, Total Carbohydrates: 3g, Fiber: 1g, Total Fat: 9g, Saturated Fat: 1g

BLACK BEAN BURGERS

VEGETARIAN | GLUTEN-FREE | NUT-FREE | SOY-FREE

These black bean burgers are easy to put together and make a great main course for a vegetarian meal. Cheesy and spicy with an appealing crispy crust, they are hard to resist. Pair these burgers with a side of Sautéed Swiss Chard with Balsamic Vinegar (page 124).

SERVES 4

Prep time: 5 minutes
Cook time: 10 minutes

2 (15-ounce) cans black beans, rinsed and drained
1 (5-ounce) can sliced jalapeño peppers, drained
½ cup shredded Cheddar cheese
¼ cup gluten-free bread crumbs
1 teaspoon ground turmeric
2 teaspoons coconut oil, divided

Ingredient Tip: Substitute 2 to 3 sliced and seeded fresh jalapeño peppers for the canned variety, if desired. Jalapeños harvested in the winter tend to be milder than those harvested in the summer, so be sure to try them first to determine the heat level (reduce the quantity if you find them too spicy).

1. In a large bowl, using a potato masher, mash the black beans. Add the jalapeños, Cheddar cheese, bread crumbs, and turmeric, and stir well.

2. Using your hands, form the mixture into 8 small patties, pressing firmly so they stay together.

3. In a large skillet, heat 1 teaspoon of oil. Working in 2 batches, cook the patties for 2 minutes per side until browned and crisp. Transfer the cooked patties to a plate lined with paper towel and repeat with the remaining coconut oil and patties. Serve immediately.

PER SERVING: Calories: 583, Protein: 31g, Cholesterol: 15mg, Sodium: 175mg, Total Carbohydrates: 97g, Fiber: 27g, Total Fat: 11g, Saturated Fat: 6g

VEGETABLE FRIED RICE

VEGETARIAN | DAIRY-FREE | NUT-FREE | LOW-FODMAP

Carrot, bell pepper, and bok choy make this classic dish suitable for Phase 1. If you are gluten intolerant, be sure to use tamari instead of soy sauce, as soy sauce is made using wheat koji and is therefore not gluten-free.

SERVES 4

Prep time: 15 minutes
Cook time: 25 minutes

2 cups water
1½ cups short-grain white or
    brown rice
3 teaspoons extra virgin olive oil,
    divided
2 eggs, beaten
Pinch asafetida
1 red bell pepper, seeded and diced
1 large carrot, peeled and
    finely diced
1 small head bok choy, cut into
    thin strips
1 tablespoon peeled fresh
    ginger, minced
3 tablespoons soy sauce
1 tablespoon rice vinegar
2 teaspoons toasted sesame oil

Variation Tip: Cold rice is preferable when making fried rice to prevent it from becoming sticky. If you have some on hand, skip step 1 and add 3 cups cold cooked rice to the pan in step 4.

1. In a small pot, combine the water and rice and bring to a boil. Reduce the heat to low, cover, and cook for 6 to 12 minutes (depending on the type of rice; follow the package directions) until all the liquid has been absorbed. Using a fork, fluff the cooked rice. Spread the rice evenly over a baking sheet. Refrigerate until needed.

2. In a large skillet or wok over medium-high heat, heat 1 teaspoon of olive oil. Pour in the beaten eggs and cook for less than 1 minute just until they begin to set. Transfer to a small bowl.

3. To the same skillet or wok over medium-high heat, heat the remaining 2 teaspoons of olive oil. Add the asafetida and cook for about 10 seconds just until fragrant. Add the bell pepper, carrot, bok choy, and ginger. Cook for 2 to 3 minutes, stirring constantly until the vegetables are just slightly tender.

4. Fold in the cooled rice.

5. Gently stir in the soy sauce and rice vinegar.

6. Fold in the cooked eggs. Remove the pan from the heat, and drizzle the fried rice with the sesame oil. Serve hot.

PER SERVING: Calories: 372, Protein: 10g, Cholesterol: 82mg, Sodium: 762mg, Total Carbohydrates: 62g, Fiber: 3g, Total Fat: 9g, Saturated Fat: 2g

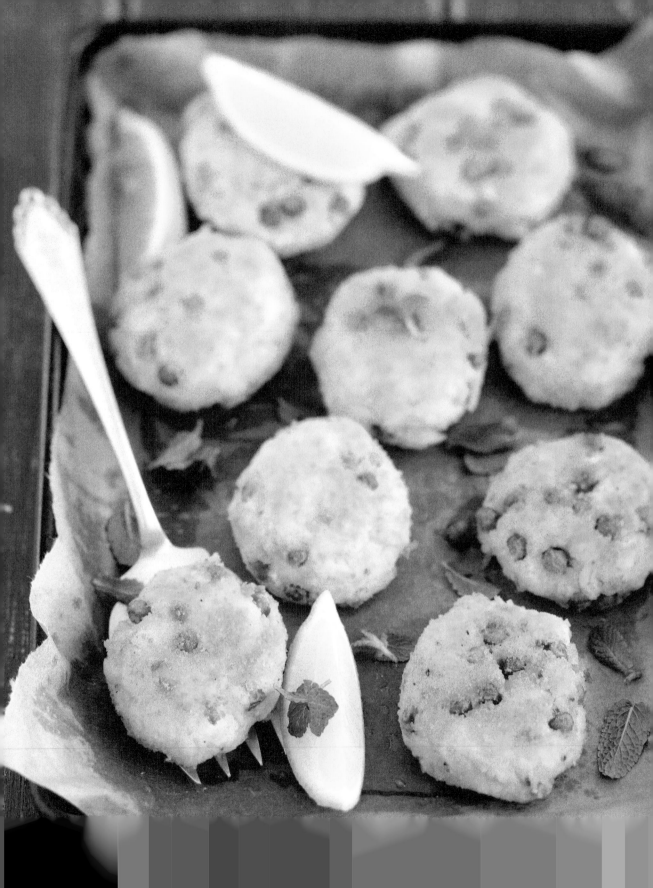

FISH & SEAFOOD

If you are a lover of fish and seafood, you'll be happy to hear that the Microbiome Diet contains plenty of these delicious foods. Make fish patties, fish pie, fish curries, or simple baked fish—there is something here for everyone. If you are not already keen on fish, you may just change your mind after trying a few of these flavorful dishes.

SALMON SALAD LETTUCE WRAPS

GRAIN-FREE | GLUTEN-FREE | NUT-FREE | SOY-FREE | LOW-FODMAP

Perfect for a light lunch or dinner, this salad is creamy and rich with just the right amount of crunch from the fresh cucumber and bell pepper, not to mention the lettuce leaf wraps. Hardboiled eggs add even more protein and keep you feeling fuller longer. This is a great way to use up leftover cooked salmon. See the Tip for cooking instructions.

SERVES 4

Prep time: 15 minutes

2 cups flaked, cooked salmon
2 hardboiled eggs, peeled and diced
1 red bell pepper, finely diced
1 cucumber, peeled, seeded,
    and diced
3 tablespoons mayonnaise
¼ teaspoon cayenne pepper
Sea salt
Freshly ground black pepper
2 tablespoons fresh lemon juice
8 large lettuce leaves

Ingredient Tip: Two cups of flaked, cooked salmon equals about 1 pound of fresh salmon fillet. Cook the salmon in a 350°F oven until the fish flakes apart easily (depending on the thickness of the salmon fillet, this could take 12 to 20 minutes). Let the fish cool slightly before proceeding with the recipe.

1. In a medium bowl, mix the salmon and eggs.

2. In a small bowl, stir together the bell pepper, cucumber, mayonnaise, and cayenne pepper. Season to taste with sea salt and pepper. Gently stir the mayonnaise mixture into the salmon and eggs. Add the lemon juice and mix well.

3. Divide the salad evenly among the lettuce leaves and roll to enclose. Serve cold.

PER SERVING: Calories: 174, Protein: 15g, Cholesterol: 110mg, Sodium: 256mg, Total Carbohydrates: 8g, Fiber: 1g, Total Fat: 10g, Saturated Fat: 2g

SALMON WITH MISO SAUCE

NUT-FREE | LOW-FODMAP

The perfect dish for surprise dinner guests, this showstopper can be ready in minutes. Red miso, which benefits from a longer fermentation period than white or yellow miso, adds rich flavor (the miso is added to a slightly cooled mixture so its live cultures can survive). The leftover sauce can be used as a salad dressing or drizzled over roasted vegetables.

SERVES 4

Prep time: 5 minutes
Cook time: 15 minutes

1 (20-ounce) skin-on salmon fillet
¼ cup whipping (35 percent) cream
2 tablespoons extra virgin olive oil
2 tablespoons rice vinegar
1 tablespoon soy sauce
1 tablespoon pure maple syrup
1 tablespoon grainy Dijon mustard
2 tablespoons red miso paste

Ingredient Tip: To make this dish gluten free, substitute gluten-free tamari for the soy sauce.

1. Preheat the oven to 425°F.

2. Line a baking sheet with parchment paper.

3. Place the salmon, skin-side down, on the prepared sheet. Bake in the preheated oven for 12 to 15 minutes until the thickest part of the salmon can be flaked apart with a fork.

4. In a small saucepan over medium heat, whisk together the whipping cream, olive oil, rice vinegar, soy sauce, maple syrup, and Dijon mustard and bring to a boil. Remove from the heat and set aside to cool slightly.

5. Just before serving, whisk the red miso paste into the sauce. Pour over individual portions of salmon and serve immediately.

PER SERVING: Calories: 309, Protein: 29g, Cholesterol: 71mg, Sodium: 656mg, Total Carbohydrates: 6g, Fiber: <1g, Total Fat: 19g, Saturated Fat: 4g

TURMERIC CURRIED SALMON

DAIRY-FREE | GRAIN-FREE | GLUTEN-FREE | NUT-FREE | SOY-FREE |
KID-FRIENDLY | LOW-FODMAP

This may be one of the simplest main course recipes in this book. Prominently featuring turmeric, an anti-inflammatory spice, this brightly colored dish is loaded with healthy omega-3 fatty acids and heaps of flavor.

SERVES 4

Prep time: 5 minutes, plus
  30 minutes chilling
Cook time: 10 minutes

1 teaspoon sea salt
1 teaspoon ground turmeric
Pinch asafetida
1 (1-pound) boneless skinless
    salmon fillet
2 teaspoons coconut oil
½ cup unsweetened coconut milk
½ teaspoon coarsely crushed
    black peppercorns

Variation Tip: This curry can also be made with any whitefish such as cod or tilapia, as well as with shrimp or scallops, for an equally pleasing and simple meal (adjust the cooking times accordingly).

1. In a small bowl, mix the sea salt, turmeric, and asafetida. Sprinkle over the top of the salmon, and use your hands to press the mixture firmly onto the flesh. Cover and refrigerate for 30 minutes, or as long as overnight.

2. In a large skillet over medium-high heat, heat the coconut oil. Add the salmon, flesh-side down, and cook for about 2 minutes until browned. Flip, and cook for about 2 minutes more until the other side is browned.

3. Add the coconut milk and crushed peppercorns. Using the spatula, lift up the salmon to allow the coconut milk to flow under the fish. Reduce the heat to medium-low, cover the pan, and cook for 3 to 5 minutes until the fish flakes easily with a fork and is cooked through.

4. Transfer the salmon to a platter and top with the pan sauce. Serve.

PER SERVING: Calories: 241, Protein: 23g, Cholesterol: 50mg, Sodium: 523mg, Total Carbohydrates: 2g, Fiber: <1g, Total Fat: 17g, Saturated Fat: 9g

SALMON PATTIES

DAIRY-FREE | GRAIN-FREE | GLUTEN-FREE | NUT-FREE | SOY-FREE |
KID-FRIENDLY | LOW-FODMAP

Serve these patties with a salad or other vegetable of your choice, and you will have a nutrient-rich meal on the table in under 30 minutes. Canned salmon delivers convenience and a rich dose of essential fatty acids. You can either pick out the larger bones from the canned salmon before mixing and shaping the patties, or leave them in, as they are a great source of calcium.

SERVES 4

Prep time: 10 minutes
Cook time: 10 minutes

---

1 (15-ounce) can wild-caught
    Alaskan salmon

3 eggs

¼ cup coconut flour

2 tablespoons chopped fresh dill

2 tablespoons chopped fresh basil

Zest of 1 lemon

1 tablespoon coconut oil

Lemon wedges, for
    serving (optional)

Phase 2 Tip: Add ½ cup fresh or frozen sweet peas to the patties in step 2.

Variation Tip: If you prefer, you can make these using fresh salmon. To do so, bake the salmon in a 350°F oven until it flakes easily with a fork (the cook time will depend on the size of the fillet). Break the cooked salmon into pieces and continue making the patties as directed in step 2.

1. Using a fine-mesh strainer, drain the salmon, pressing down with a spoon to remove as much moisture as possible. Transfer the salmon to a mixing bowl.

2. Add the eggs, coconut flour, dill, basil, and lemon zest. Stir well. Using your hands, shape the mixture into 4 patties.

3. In a large skillet over medium-high heat, heat the coconut oil. Cook the salmon patties for 2 to 3 minutes per side until golden brown. Serve hot with lemon wedges on the side (if using).

PER SERVING: Calories: 257, Protein: 36g, Cholesterol: 170mg, Sodium: 98mg, Total Carbohydrates: 3g, Fiber: 1g, Total Fat: 17g, Saturated Fat: 8g

SALMON BAKED WITH HERBS

DAIRY-FREE | GRAIN-FREE | GLUTEN-FREE | NUT-FREE | SOY-FREE | KID-FRIENDLY

If you are a salmon lover, you will really enjoy this simple and flavorful preparation. Scallions and parsley lend an herbal flavor to the fish. Serve with a salad, Cauliflower Rice (see page 133), or your favorite side dish.

SERVES 4

Prep time: 10 minutes, plus
   15 minutes marinating
Cook time: 12 minutes, plus
   10 minutes resting

1¼ pounds boneless skinless
   salmon fillets
Sea salt
Freshly cracked black pepper
2 tablespoons extra virgin olive oil
Juice of 2 lemons
½ cup chopped scallions (green
   part only)
½ cup chopped fresh flat-leaf Italian
   parsley leaves
¼ cup dry white wine
2 lemons, cut into wedges,
   for garnish

Variation Tip: Before baking the fish in step 4, sprinkle with ½ cup of grated Parmesan cheese.

1. Preheat the oven to 425°F.

2. Place the salmon in a baking dish and season well with sea salt and pepper.

3. In a small bowl, whisk together the olive oil and lemon juice. Pour over the salmon. Let sit at room temperature for 15 minutes.

4. Arrange the scallions and parsley evenly over the top of and underneath the salmon. Pour the white wine into the baking dish, beside the fish. Bake in the preheated oven for 12 minutes until nearly cooked through (insert the tip of a knife to check doneness; there should be only a bit of uncooked flesh at the thickest part of the fillet).

5. Remove the dish from the oven and cover with aluminum foil. Let sit for 10 minutes (the residual heat will finish cooking the fish).

6. Divide the fish into 4 servings. Garnish with lemon wedges and serve immediately.

PER SERVING: Calories: 270, Protein: 28g, Cholesterol: 63mg, Sodium: 306mg, Total Carbohydrates: 2g, Fiber: <1g, Total Fat: 16g, Saturated Fat: 2g

TUNA & QUINOA PATTIES

GLUTEN-FREE | NUT-FREE | SOY-FREE | LOW-FODMAP

Quinoa is so versatile. Here it adds protein and texture to simple tuna patties. A little Parmesan cheese adds a nice savory edge. Serve these on their own or on top of a simple green salad for a complete meal.

SERVES 4

Prep time: 10 minutes
Cook time: 25 minutes

1 cup quinoa, rinsed and drained
2 cups Vegetable Stock (page 99)
    or water
1 (5-ounce) can tuna packed in water
2 eggs, lightly beaten
½ teaspoon freshly ground
    black pepper
½ teaspoon sea salt
¼ cup grated Parmesan cheese
2 teaspoons extra virgin olive oil

Ingredient Tip: Quinoa can be cooked in advance for later use. Refrigerate cooked quinoa in an airtight container for up to 5 days. For even easier prep, prepare quinoa in a rice cooker (follow the manufacturer's instructions).

1. In a small saucepan over medium-high heat, combine the quinoa and vegetable stock and bring to a boil. Cover, reduce the heat to low, and simmer for 10 to 15 minutes until all the liquid is absorbed. Fluff the cooked quinoa with a fork and set aside to cool.

2. In a medium bowl, stir together the tuna, beaten eggs, black pepper, sea salt, and Parmesan cheese until well combined. Mix in the cooled quinoa.

3. In a large skillet over medium heat, heat the olive oil. Using your hands, form the mixture into patties (about ⅓ cup for each). Add to the hot oil and cook for 2 to 3 minutes per side until browned. Take care when flipping, as the patties will be crumbly until cooked and set. Serve hot.

PER SERVING: Calories: 317, Protein: 23g, Cholesterol: 98mg, Sodium: 732mg, Total Carbohydrates: 28g, Fiber: 3g, Total Fat: 12g, Saturated Fat: 3g

BROILED SOLE WITH ORANGE, WHITE WINE & DILL

DAIRY-FREE | GRAIN-FREE | GLUTEN-FREE | NUT-FREE | SOY-FREE

Sole is a great fish for broiling because it is typically thin and, therefore, cooks quickly. White wine adds a touch of acidity and fruitiness to this quick preparation, so don't skip it (the alcohol burns off during cooking).

SERVES 4

Prep time: 5 minutes
Cook time: 25 minutes

¾ cup dry white wine
¼ teaspoon dried dill
1 pound skinless boneless sole fillets
1 teaspoon extra virgin olive oil
Sea salt
Freshly ground black pepper
1 orange, sliced

Variation Tip: Substitute tilapia or Arctic char for the sole (adjust the cooking time accordingly).

1. In a small saucepan, combine the white wine and dill and bring to a boil. Reduce the heat to low and simmer for 15 to 20 minutes until the wine is reduced by about half. Cover and set aside.

2. Preheat the broiler to high, placing a rack 5 to 6 inches from the top. Line a baking sheet with aluminum foil.

3. Rub both sides of the fish with olive oil and season to taste with sea salt and pepper. Place the fish on the prepared sheet and top with the orange slices. Broil for about 5 minutes, or until the fish turns opaque and flakes easily with a fork.

4. Transfer the cooked fish to a serving plate and top with the reserved sauce.

PER SERVING: Calories: 188, Protein: 26g, Cholesterol: 7g, Sodium: 325mg, Total Carbohydrates: 7g, Fiber: 1g, Total Fat: 2g, Saturated Fat: 0g

WHITEFISH CAKES

GLUTEN-FREE | NUT-FREE | SOY-FREE | LOW-FODMAP

Tuna and salmon may be the obvious favorites for fish cakes, but whitefish works beautifully, as well. Seasoned with mustard, paprika, red pepper flakes, and mayonnaise, these tilapia cakes make an elegant and filling main course.

SERVES 4

Prep time: 5 minutes, plus
   30 minutes chilling
Cook time: 10 to 20 minutes

---

2 teaspoons extra virgin olive oil
1 pound boneless skinless
   tilapia fillets
⅓ cup mayonnaise
⅓ cup gluten-free bread crumbs
1 large egg
1 large egg yolk
1 teaspoon mustard powder
1 teaspoon sea salt
½ teaspoon dried parsley
¼ teaspoon freshly cracked
   black pepper
¼ teaspoon sweet paprika
¼ teaspoon red pepper flakes
1½ tablespoons butter

Ingredient Tip: Look for gluten-free bread crumbs in the natural food section of well-stocked grocery stores or health food stores. Alternatively, you can make your own gluten-free bread crumbs by processing crispy brown rice cereal, gluten-free pretzels, or rice cereal squares in a food processor.

1. In a large skillet over medium-high heat, heat the olive oil. Add the tilapia and cook for 3 to 5 minutes per side until the fish is opaque and flakes easily with a fork. Transfer to a plate to cool. Once cool, flake the cooked fish with a fork.

2. In a large bowl, combine the flaked fish, mayonnaise, bread crumbs, egg, egg yolk, mustard powder, sea salt, parsley, pepper, paprika, and red pepper flakes. Using your hands, shape the mixture into 6 to 8 small patties and place on a baking sheet. Refrigerate for 30 minutes so the patties firm up.

3. In a large skillet over medium heat, melt the butter. Working in batches, cook the patties for 3 to 5 minutes per side until browned. Repeat with any remaining patties. Serve hot.

PER SERVING: Calories: 297, Protein: 25g, Cholesterol: 165mg, Sodium: 760mg, Total Carbohydrates: 12g, Fiber: <1g, Total Fat: 17g, Saturated Fat: 5g

WHOLE ROASTED MACKEREL

DAIRY-FREE | GRAIN-FREE | GLUTEN-FREE | NUT-FREE | SOY-FREE | LOW-FODMAP

If you've never cooked a whole fish before, you'll be thrilled with this easy preparation—it's quick and delicious. Mackerel is a sustainable fish loaded with omega-3 fatty acids.

SERVES 4

Prep time: 5 minutes
Cook time: 25 minutes

---

1 (2- to 3-pound) whole mackerel, scaled, gutted, and gills removed (ask your fishmonger to do this for you)
2 tablespoons extra virgin olive oil
Sea salt
Freshly cracked black pepper
1 lemon, sliced
¼ cup chopped fresh flat-leaf Italian parsley leaves
1 lemon, cut into wedges, for garnish

Ingredient Tip: When shopping for mackerel, look for a fish with bright clear eyes and shiny skin. It should not smell fishy, and the gills should appear clean. Because fresh mackerel spoils quickly, it is often sold frozen. To thaw frozen mackerel, place it in a covered container in the refrigerator overnight.

1. Preheat the oven to 475°F and position a rack in the middle of the oven.

2. Line a baking sheet with parchment paper.

3. Place the fish on the prepared baking sheet. Drizzle with the olive oil and, using your hands, rub it all over the outside of the fish. Season the fish to taste, inside and outside, with sea salt and pepper. Stuff the lemon slices and parsley into the cavity of the fish.

4. Bake in the preheated oven for 20 to 25 minutes until cooked through (when the fish is cooked, its eyes will turn white, its body will be firm to the touch, and the flesh will flake easily with a fork). Serve on a platter, garnished with the lemon wedges.

PER SERVING: Calories: 659, Protein: 54g, Cholesterol: 170mg, Sodium: 427mg, Total Carbohydrates: <1g, Fiber: 0g, Total Fat: 48g, Saturated Fat: 11g

SMOKED MACKEREL, POTATO & ARUGULA SALAD

DAIRY-FREE | GRAIN-FREE | GLUTEN-FREE | NUT-FREE | SOY-FREE

Smoked mackerel, which is ready to eat, minimizes the work you must do to enjoy this simple salad. Fingerling potatoes are small and quick cooking, and lend a buttery texture. Served on a bed of arugula, which is rich in vitamins A and C, folic acid, and calcium, this is a well-rounded salad with loads of flavor.

SERVES 4

Prep time: 15 minutes
Cook time: 20 minutes

1 pound fingerling potatoes
2 tablespoons extra virgin olive oil
1 tablespoon red wine vinegar
1 teaspoon whole-grain mustard
Sea salt
Freshly cracked black pepper
1 (9-ounce) can smoked
    mackerel, flaked
4 cups arugula leaves
Lemon wedges, for garnish

Ingredient Tip: Arugula is in season in early summer and fall. Look for it at farmers' markets or any well-stocked grocery store. Or, if you have a little gardening space, grow a patch yourself. It is quite easy to grow and one of the first salad crops of the season, thriving in cool spring weather.

1. In a saucepan, cover the potatoes with water and bring to a boil. Cook for 15 to 20 minutes, until tender. Drain and set aside to cool.

2. In a large bowl, whisk together the olive oil, red wine vinegar, and mustard. Set aside.

3. Cut the cooled potatoes in half and add to the bowl with the dressing. Toss until well coated. Season to taste with sea salt and pepper. Fold in the flaked mackerel.

4. Divide the arugula evenly among 4 serving plates. Top each serving with an equal amount of mackerel and potato salad. Serve garnished with lemon wedges.

PER SERVING: Calories: 316, Protein: 18g, Cholesterol: 48mg, Sodium: 299mg, Total Carbohydrates: 19g, Fiber: 2g, Total Fat: 19mg, Saturated Fat: 4g

MEDITERRANEAN BAKED WHITEFISH

DAIRY-FREE | GRAIN-FREE | GLUTEN-FREE | NUT-FREE | SOY-FREE | LOW-FODMAP

With a combination of olives, tomatoes, and wine, this fish dish is one you don't want to miss. Simple, with minimal prep for a weeknight, you can have this on the table in about 30 minutes. If you can't find halibut, try cod, haddock, or striped bass.

SERVES 4

Prep time: 5 minutes
Cook time: 20 minutes

1 pound halibut fillets
Sea salt
Freshly cracked black pepper
1 tablespoon extra virgin olive oil
Pinch asafetida
2 cups diced tomatoes, with juice
½ cup pitted Kalamata olives
2 tablespoons dry white wine
1 teaspoon dried basil leaves
¼ teaspoon dried thyme leaves

Time-Saving Tip: Keep a few cans of diced tomatoes on hand at all times—there are so many things you can make with them. For this recipe one (15-ounce) can of tomatoes is roughly equivalent to 2 cups of fresh diced tomatoes.

1. Preheat the oven to 375°F.

2. Line a baking dish with parchment paper.

3. Place the fish in the prepared baking dish, and season lightly with sea salt and pepper. Bake in the preheated oven for 12 to 15 minutes until the fish is nearly cooked through. Remove from the oven and set aside.

4. In a small saucepan over medium heat, heat the olive oil. Add the asafetida and cook for about 20 seconds, stirring constantly until fragrant.

5. Stir in the tomatoes, olives, white wine, basil, and thyme. Bring the mixture to a simmer and cook for 3 minutes until heated through and the flavors have melded.

6. Pour the tomato sauce over the fish. Return the pan to the oven and bake for 5 minutes more, until the fish is cooked through and flakes easily with a fork.

PER SERVING: Calories: 191, Protein: 27g, Cholesterol: 62mg, Sodium: 474mg, Total Carbohydrates: 5g, Fiber: 2g, Total Fat: 7g, Saturated Fat: 1g

CURRIED COCONUT WHITEFISH

GRAIN-FREE | GLUTEN-FREE | NUT-FREE | SOY-FREE | LOW-FODMAP

Curry is a warming spice blend with so many uses in the kitchen. Here, it lends a beautiful flavoring to sole, which is then coated in coconut shreds and baked to perfection. Dip this mild fish in its accompanying cooling yogurt-cilantro sauce, and you have a satisfying meal that manages to include a little probiotic goodness.

SERVES 4

Prep time: 10 minutes
Cook time: 10 minutes, plus
  2 minutes resting

½ cup plain yogurt (not fat-free)
2 tablespoons chopped fresh
  cilantro leaves
Sea salt
Freshly ground black pepper
1 tablespoon curry powder
1 pound skinless boneless sole fillets
2 large egg whites
1 cup dried unsweetened
  shredded coconut

Ingredient Tip: Curry powders vary considerably by brand. Check the label to ensure that your curry powder does not contain garlic.

1. Preheat the oven to 500°F.

2. Line a baking sheet with parchment paper.

3. In a small bowl, mix the yogurt and cilantro. Season to taste with sea salt and pepper. Set aside.

4. Sprinkle the curry powder over the fish, and use your fingers to rub it into the flesh on both sides.

5. Set up a breading station: In a shallow bowl, whisk the egg whites until foamy. In another shallow bowl, place the dried coconut.

6. Dip the fillets in the egg whites and then roll in the coconut. Arrange in a single layer on the prepared sheet, and season to taste with sea salt and pepper.

7. Bake in the preheated oven for 8 to 10 minutes until the fish is opaque and flakes easily with a fork. Remove from the oven and set aside for 2 minutes.

8. Serve with the yogurt sauce on the side.

PER SERVING: Calories: 226, Protein: 30g, Cholesterol: 64mg, Sodium: 366mg, Total Carbohydrates: 6g, Fiber: 2g, Total Fat: 8g, Saturated Fat: 7g

THAI-STYLE WHITEFISH SALAD

DAIRY-FREE | GRAIN-FREE | NUT-FREE | LOW-FODMAP

Balancing the salty, spicy, and sour elements that Thai cuisine is known for, this dish is quick to prepare, nourishing, and delicious. Bean sprouts are easy to digest and contain high levels of vitamin B and C vitamins. Feel free to substitute your favorite whitefish, such as halibut, rockfish, sole, or pollock as available seasonally.

SERVES 4

Prep time: 10 minutes
Cook time: 10 minutes

For the dressing
1 red Thai chile, seeded and
     finely diced
¼ cup soy sauce
Juice of 2 limes
1 tablespoon pure maple syrup

For the salad
2 heads red or green leaf lettuce,
     torn or cut into bite-size pieces
2 cups bean sprouts
1 bunch fresh cilantro, leaves
     removed and chopped
1 large tomato, diced
2 teaspoons extra virgin olive oil
1 pound cod fillets
Sea salt
Freshly cracked black pepper

Substitution Tip: If you adhere to a gluten-free diet, be sure to choose a gluten-free soy sauce, such as tamari, to avoid traces of wheat. If fish is an allergen, use chicken breast (see page 113) shredded over the salad in place of the fish.

To make the dressing
In a small bowl, whisk together the chile, soy sauce, lime juice, and maple syrup. Set aside.

To make the salad
1. In a large bowl, place the lettuce. Add the bean sprouts, cilantro, and tomatoes. Toss to combine.

2. Season the fish with sea salt and pepper.

3. In a large skillet over medium-high heat, heat the olive oil. Add the fish and cook for 3 to 5 minutes per side, or until the fish is cooked through and flakes easily with a fork.

4. Divide the salad among 4 plates. Top each plate with a portion of fish and drizzle with the soy-lime dressing. Serve.

PER SERVING: Calories: 205, Protein: 31g, Cholesterol: 62mg, Sodium: 1,236mg, Total Carbohydrates: 12g, Fiber: 1g, Total Fat: 4g, Saturated Fat: <1g

CRUNCHY OVEN-BAKED WHITEFISH

DAIRY-FREE | GLUTEN-FREE | NUT-FREE | SOY-FREE | KID-FRIENDLY | LOW-FODMAP

Using gluten-free bread crumbs, you can create "fried" fish the healthier way—in the oven. Simply bread the fish as you would for frying, pop them in the oven for about 20 minutes, and dinner is ready. Pair these fillets with a salad and be sure to have some Tartar Sauce (page 226) on hand.

SERVES 4

Prep time: 10 minutes
Cook time: 20 to 30 minutes

1 teaspoon extra virgin olive oil
2 cups gluten-free bread crumbs
2 eggs, beaten
1 pound cod fillets or other whitefish
Sea salt
Freshly cracked black pepper

Substitution Tip: If fish is an allergen, or just for something different, this method of breading can also be used for chicken. Use boneless skinless chicken thighs for the most flavorful and juicy meat, or chicken breast strips, and follow the recipe directions.

1. Preheat the oven 350°F.

2. Line a baking sheet with aluminum foil and spread the olive oil evenly over the sheet.

3. Arrange the gluten-free bread crumbs on a large plate. Place the beaten eggs in a small bowl.

4. Season the fish to taste with sea salt and pepper. Dip the fish into the egg mixture, shaking off any excess. Roll the fish in the bread crumbs, pressing down to encourage as much as possible to stick to the fish. Arrange the fish on the prepared sheet.

5. Bake in the preheated oven for 20 to 30 minutes, until cooked through and browned, flipping once halfway through. Serve hot.

PER SERVING: Calories: 374, Protein: 36g, Cholesterol: 144mg, Sodium: 749mg, Total Carbohydrates: 31g, Fiber: 2g, Total Fat: 7g, Saturated Fat: 2g

EASY FISH PIE

GRAIN-FREE | GLUTEN-FREE | NUT-FREE | SOY-FREE

If you love shepherd's pie made with chicken or beef, then you are bound to enjoy this lighter take on the classic dish. Made with a mild-tasting whitefish, this pie bursts with flavor and is a time-tested comfort food at its finest. Prepare the dish the night before and pop it in the oven for dinnertime.

SERVES 4

Prep time: 15 minutes
Cook time: 1 hour

2 pounds russet potatoes, peeled and diced
2 cups roughly chopped fresh spinach leaves
1 carrot, peeled and grated
1 small rutabaga, peeled and grated
¼ cup chopped fresh flat-leaf Italian parsley leaves
Zest of 1 lemon
Juice of 1 lemon
½ pound boneless skinless salmon fillet, cut into bite-size pieces
½ pound boneless skinless sole fillet, cut into bite-size pieces
2 tablespoons extra virgin olive oil, divided
Sea salt
Freshly ground black pepper
1 cup shredded Cheddar cheese

Variation Tip: Add 1 cup of corn or sweet peas to the pie in step 3.

1. Preheat the oven 400°F.

2. In a large pot over medium-high heat, cover the potatoes with salted water and bring to a boil. Reduce the heat to low and simmer for 10 to 15 minutes until tender. Use a knife or fork to test for doneness.

3. In a large bowl, place the spinach, carrot, rutabaga, parsley, and lemon zest. Toss to combine.

4. Add the salmon and sole to the vegetables. Squeeze the lemon juice over the mixture and stir to combine. Add 1 tablespoon of olive oil and toss to combine.

5. Drain the potatoes and return them to the pot. Using a potato masher, mash them well. Add the remaining tablespoon of olive oil and season to taste with sea salt and pepper.

6. Transfer the fish and vegetables to a pie dish, pressing down to fill the dish. Top with the mashed potatoes and sprinkle with Cheddar cheese.

7. Bake in the preheated oven for 45 minutes until the fish is cooked through and the top is nicely browned.

PER SERVING: Calories: 515, Protein: 37g, Cholesterol: 86mg, Sodium: 540mg, Total Carbohydrates: 46g, Fiber: 9g, Total Fat: 21g, Saturated Fat: 8g

COCONUT SHRIMP

DAIRY-FREE | GLUTEN-FREE | NUT-FREE | SOY-FREE | KID-FRIENDLY | LOW-FODMAP

These baked coconut shrimp are crisp and slightly sweet—just be sure to use unsweetened coconut. Serve with Tartar Sauce (page 226), or on its own with a salad or roasted vegetables for a light meal.

SERVES 4

Prep time: 10 minutes
Cook time: 10 minutes

Cooking spray
1 pound large raw shrimp, peeled
    and deveined
Sea salt
1 egg
½ cup gluten-free bread crumbs
½ cup unsweetened
    shredded coconut

Variation Tip: Add even more flavor by seasoning the shrimp with a Cajun seasoning or other flavored seasoning blend. However, be sure to adjust the amount of salt you add, as many types of flavored seasonings contain salt.

1. Preheat the oven 425°F.

2. Line a baking sheet with aluminum foil and spray with nonstick cooking spray.

3. Season the shrimp with sea salt.

4. Set up a breading station: In a shallow bowl, lightly beat the egg with a fork. In another bowl, mix the bread crumbs and coconut.

5. Dip the seasoned shrimp into the egg and then roll in the bread crumbs. Transfer the breaded shrimp to the prepared sheet.

6. Bake in the preheated oven for 5 minutes, turn the shrimp over, and bake for 5 minutes more until browned and crisp.

PER SERVING: Calories: 239, Protein: 29g, Cholesterol: 280mg, Sodium: 627mg, Total Carbohydrates: 13g, Fiber: 2g, Total Fat: 7g, Saturated Fat: 4g

LEMON SHRIMP

GRAIN-FREE | GLUTEN-FREE | NUT-FREE | SOY-FREE | KID-FRIENDLY | LOW-FODMAP

If you love shrimp scampi, but think it can't be done without garlic, think again. This simple dish is reinvented with a mixture of lemon, parsley, and a sprinkling of Parmesan cheese.

SERVES 4

Prep time: 10 minutes
Cook time: 10 minutes

2 tablespoons extra virgin olive oil
1 tablespoon butter
¼ cup dry white wine
¼ cup fresh lemon juice
½ teaspoon dried oregano
½ teaspoon sea salt
¼ teaspoon freshly cracked
   black pepper
1 pound large raw shrimp, peeled
   and deveined
¼ cup chopped fresh flat-leaf Italian
   parsley leaves
¼ cup grated Parmesan cheese

Substitution Tip: If desired, clarified butter or ghee can be substituted for the butter, or it can be omitted altogether. If you omit the butter, increase the amount of olive oil to 3 tablespoons.

1. In a large skillet over medium-high heat, heat the olive oil and butter. Sir in the white wine, lemon juice, oregano, sea salt, and pepper.

2. Add the shrimp and cook for 5 to 7 minutes, stirring often until the shrimp turn pink. Sprinkle with the parsley and continue to cook for 2 minutes more, stirring.

3. Remove the pan from the heat and add the Parmesan cheese. Let the shrimp sit for 1 or 2 minutes, until the cheese melts slightly. Serve hot over rice or Cauliflower Rice (page 133).

PER SERVING: Calories: 261, Protein: 28g, Cholesterol: 252mg, Sodium: 603mg, Total Carbohydrates: 3g, Fiber: 0mg, Total Fat: 14g, Saturated Fat: 5g

GINGER SCALLOP STIR-FRY

DAIRY-FREE | NUT-FREE | LOW-FODMAP

Brightly flavored, this dish makes a light meal when served over rice, Cauliflower Rice (page 133), or quinoa. Do not extend the marinating time beyond 10 minutes, as the scallops will begin to "cook" in the lime juice.

SERVES 4

Prep time: 10 minutes, plus
  10 minutes marinating
Cook time: 15 minutes

¼ cup fresh lime juice

¼ cup rice cooking wine

1 pound bay scallops

¼ cup cold water

2 tablespoons rice starch

2 tablespoons sesame oil

1 red bell pepper, diced

1-inch piece peeled fresh
    ginger, minced

¼ cup sliced scallions (green
    part only)

¼ cup soy sauce

Ingredient Tip: Find rice cooking wine in the Asian food section of well-stocked grocery stores or Asian markets. A popular variety, Shaoxing rice cooking wine, is widely available and an inexpensive choice.

1. In a nonreactive bowl, combine the lime juice and rice wine. Add the scallops and set aside for 10 minutes to marinate.

2. In a small bowl, combine the cold water and rice starch and stir well. Set aside.

3. In a wok or large skillet over medium-high heat, heat the sesame oil. Add the bell pepper and ginger, and cook for 3 minutes, stirring constantly until the ginger is fragrant and the bell pepper begins to soften. Add the scallion greens and mix well.

4. Drain the scallops (discard the marinade) and add to the wok. Cook for 3 to 5 minutes, stirring constantly until the scallops turn opaque.

5. Stir in the soy sauce. Add the rice starch-water mixture and cook for 2 to 3 minutes more, stirring constantly until the sauce thickens. Serve hot.

PER SERVING: Calories: 234, Protein: 21g, Cholesterol: 37mg, Sodium: 1,218mg, Total Carbohydrates: 20g, Fiber: 1g, Total Fat: 8g, Saturated Fat: 1g

SEA SCALLOPS WITH GREMOLATA

GRAIN-FREE | GLUTEN-FREE | NUT-FREE | SOY-FREE | LOW-FODMAP

Sea scallops are large and meaty, and loaded with protein. In this dish, a gremolata of parsley, cilantro, and lime adds an addictive bright and savory flavor.

SERVES 4

Prep time: 10 minutes, plus
10 minutes marinating
Cook time: 15 minutes

For the gremolata

½ cup finely chopped fresh flat-leaf
Italian parsley leaves
½ cup finely chopped fresh
cilantro leaves
Zest of 1 lemon
Juice of 1 lemon
½ teaspoon sea salt
½ teaspoon freshly ground
black pepper
Pinch asafetida

For the scallops

1½ pounds sea scallops
Sea salt
Freshly ground black pepper
1 tablespoon butter
1 tablespoon extra virgin olive oil

*Phase 2 Tip: In Phase 2, substitute
3 cloves of crushed garlic for
the asafetida.*

To make the gremolata

In a small bowl, stir together the parsley, cilantro, lemon juice and zest, sea salt, pepper, and asafetida. Set aside.

To make the scallops

1. Using paper towel, pat the excess moisture from the scallops. Season to taste with sea salt and pepper.

2. In a large skillet over medium-high heat, heat the butter and olive oil. Working in batches, cook half of the scallops for 2 to 3 minutes per side until browned and cooked through. Transfer to a plate and set aside. Repeat with the remaining scallops.

3. Divide the scallops evenly among 4 serving plates, and top each serving with a spoonful of gremolata.

PER SERVING: Calories: 213, Protein: 29g, Cholesterol: 64mg, Sodium: 654mg, Total Carbohydrates: 5g, Fiber: 0g, Total Fat: 8g, Saturated Fat: 3g

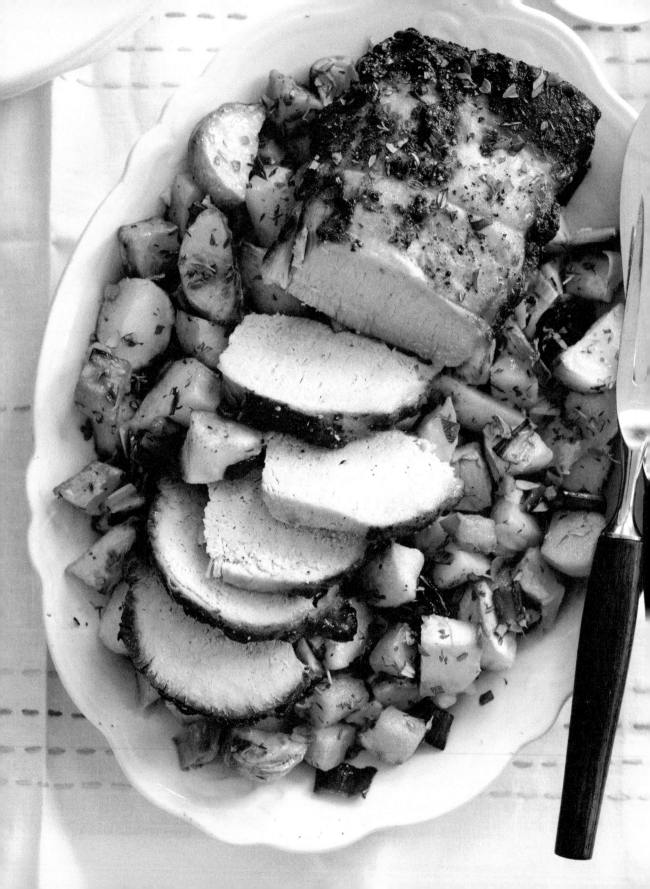

MEAT & POULTRY

These main course offerings span the gamut of cuisines, preparation styles, and flavors. It can be hard to change eating habits, but with the variety of dishes in this chapter, you won't find yourself lacking for choice. Designed to fit busy schedules, these meals require minimal prep and hands-on cooking time, making it easier to stick to the diet.

ROAST CHICKEN FOR LATER

DAIRY-FREE | GRAIN-FREE | GLUTEN-FREE | NUT-FREE | SOY-FREE |
KID-FRIENDLY | LOW-FODMAP

Several recipes in this book require cooked chicken as the main ingredient. This recipe provides an easy way to cook chicken for several meals at once so you can put some away in the refrigerator or freezer for later. For an easy, light meal, serve slices of chicken over a bed of greens with crushed walnuts and raspberry vinaigrette dressing (page 225). Bone-in chicken is used here because it is less expensive, retains more moisture, and develops a better flavor than boneless chicken breasts.

MAKES 6 TO 8 CUPS

Prep time: 5 minutes
Cook time: 45 minutes, plus
 30 minutes cooling

5 to 6 bone-in chicken breasts,
 trimmed of fat
Extra virgin olive oil
Sea salt
Freshly cracked black pepper

Variation Tip: You can save even more money by roasting a whole chicken (adjust the cooking time as needed).

1. Preheat the oven to 350°F.

2. Arrange the chicken in a large baking dish, breast-side up. Drizzle with olive oil and, using your hands, rub it all over the chicken. Season to taste with sea salt and pepper (keep in mind that this chicken will be incorporated into a larger dish, so don't overdo the salt).

3. Roast in the preheated oven for 45 minutes, or until the juices run clear. Remove from the oven and set aside to cool for 30 minutes.

4. When cool enough to handle, remove the meat from the bones (discard the skin and bones). Using a sharp knife, chop the chicken into bite-size pieces. Divide into 2-cup portions and place in freezer-safe containers. Refrigerate for up to 4 days or freeze for up to 1 month.

PER SERVING: Calories: 235, Protein: 33g, Cholesterol: 101mg, Sodium: 254mg, Total Carbohydrates: 0g, Fiber: 0g, Total Fat: 11g, Saturated Fat: 3g

CHICKEN SALAD WRAPS

GRAIN-FREE | GLUTEN-FREE | NUT-FREE | SOY-FREE | KID-FRIENDLY | LOW-FODMAP

This quick and filling lunch can be prepared in minutes. Use cooked chicken from Roast Chicken for Later (page 171) or Chicken Stock (page 100). Here, lettuce is used as a wrap, but you can also serve it in cucumber "boats" (slice an English cucumber lengthwise, scoop out the center, and fill it with chicken salad).

SERVES 4

Prep time: 10 minutes

---

2 cups diced cooked chicken

½ cup mayonnaise

2 tablespoons chopped fresh
flat-leaf Italian parsley leaves

1 teaspoon Dijon mustard

½ teaspoon sea salt

¼ teaspoon freshly ground
black pepper

8 large lettuce leaves

Phase 2 Tip: Add ¼ cup halved seedless grapes and 1 stalk of finely chopped celery to the salad in step 1.

1. In a large bowl, stir together the chicken, mayonnaise, parsley, Dijon mustard, sea salt, and pepper.

2. Divide the salad evenly among the 8 lettuce leaves. To roll the wraps, place the lettuce leaves stem side down, fold the left and right edges inward, and, starting from the bottom, roll the lettuce away from you to form a cylinder. Serve immediately.

PER SERVING: Calories: 223, Protein: 21g, Cholesterol: 62mg, Sodium: 503mg, Total Carbohydrates: 8g, Fiber: 0g, Total Fat: 12g, Saturated Fat: 2g

SEA KELP NOODLES & CHICKEN STIR-FRY

DAIRY-FREE | NUT-FREE | LOW-FODMAP

Sea kelp noodles are allergen-free and resemble traditional wheat or rice glass noodles, but have a unique texture that works well in stir-fries. You can have this nutritious stir-fry—packed with bell pepper, carrots, and broccoli—on the table in 30 minutes.

SERVES 4

Prep time: 15 minutes
Cook time: 20 minutes

2 teaspoons extra virgin olive
    oil, divided
2 large boneless skinless chicken
    breasts, cut on the bias into
    thin strips
1 red bell pepper, seeded and sliced
1 head broccoli, cut into small florets
3 medium carrots, grated
1-inch piece peeled fresh
    ginger, minced
1 (12-ounce) package kelp noodles,
    rinsed and chopped into 3- to
    4-inch pieces
3 tablespoons soy sauce
2 tablespoons fresh lime juice

Ingredient Tip: Sea kelp noodles are made of pure kelp, and are low in carbohydrates and calories. Find them at Asian markets and online.

1. In a large skillet or wok over medium-high heat, heat 1 teaspoon of olive oil. Add the chicken and cook, stirring frequently until evenly browned. Transfer the browned chicken to a plate lined with paper towels and set aside.

2. In the same skillet or wok, heat the remaining teaspoon of olive oil. Add the red bell pepper and broccoli. Sauté for about 5 minutes until just beginning to soften.

3. Add the carrots and cook for 2 to 4 minutes, stirring frequently until the vegetables begin to soften.

4. Add the ginger and cook for about 30 seconds, stirring constantly until fragrant. Return the browned chicken to the pan and stir to combine.

5. Stir in the kelp noodles, soy sauce, and lime juice. Cook for 2 to 3 minutes more, until all of the ingredients are heated through and the flavors meld. Serve hot.

PER SERVING: Calories: 244, Protein: 31g, Cholesterol: 73mg, Sodium: 1,108mg, Total Carbohydrates: 18g, Fiber: 4g, Total Fat: 6g, Saturated Fat: <1g

MISO CHICKEN & BUCKWHEAT SOBA STIR-FRY

DAIRY-FREE | NUT-FREE | KID-FRIENDLY | LOW-FODMAP

This savory Asian-influenced stir-fry is a simple fix for a busy night. To make it really stand out, marinate the chicken in the miso, vinegar, and maple syrup overnight in the refrigerator.

SERVES 4

Prep time: 15 minutes,
  plus overnight marinating
Cook time: 20 minutes

¼ cup rice vinegar

1 tablespoon white miso paste

1 tablespoon pure maple syrup

1 pound boneless skinless chicken
    breast, cubed

1 (8-ounce) package 100 percent
    buckwheat soba noodles

1 tablespoon sesame oil, divided

1-inch piece peeled fresh
    ginger, grated

1 red bell pepper, thinly sliced

1 carrot, grated

Ingredient Tip: Find 100 percent buckwheat soba noodles at well-stocked Asian markets or health food stores. Be sure to read the label, as many brands contain wheat flour. If you have no luck locally, there are many brands of pure buckwheat soba noodles available online.

1. In a small bowl or resealable bag, combine the rice vinegar, miso, and maple syrup. Add the chicken and turn to coat. Cover or seal, and refrigerate overnight.

2. In a large pot of boiling water, cook the soba noodles according to the package directions. Drain and rinse under cool running water.

3. In a large skillet or wok over medium-high heat, heat 2 teaspoons of sesame oil. Remove the chicken from the marinade (discard the marinade) and add it to the skillet. Cook for 5 to 6 minutes until browned. Transfer the cooked chicken to a plate lined with paper towel and set aside.

4. In the same skillet or wok, heat the remaining 1 teaspoon of sesame oil. Add the ginger and cook for about 30 seconds until just fragrant.

5. Add the bell pepper and carrot, and cook for 2 to 3 minutes, stirring constantly. Transfer to the plate with the chicken.

6. To the skillet, add the cooked noodles. Cook for 2 to 3 minutes, stirring frequently until heated through.

7. Return the chicken and vegetables to the skillet and cook, stirring frequently just to heat through. Serve.

PER SERVING: Calories: 454, Protein: 46g, Cholesterol: 97mg, Sodium: 752mg, Total Carbohydrates: 50g, Fiber: 1g, Total Fat: 8g, Saturated Fat: <1g

PEANUT-GINGER CHICKEN SOBA NOODLES

KID-FRIENDLY | LOW-FODMAP

Ginger is a warming spice that stimulates digestion, and its anti-inflammatory properties promote healing. It also marries well with the chicken and peanuts in this dish. If you prefer some heat, add a little more chili paste to suit your taste.

SERVES 4

Prep time: 15 minutes
Cook time: 10 minutes

⅓ cup chunky peanut butter

¼ cup soy sauce

2 tablespoons rice vinegar

2 tablespoons pure maple syrup

1 teaspoon Asian-style chili paste

1-inch piece peeled fresh ginger, roughly chopped

1 or 2 tablespoons water

1 tablespoon sea salt

1 (8-ounce) package 100 percent buckwheat soba noodles

2 tablespoons sesame oil

2 cups cooked chopped chicken (see Roast Chicken for Later, page 171)

¼ cup chopped scallions (green part only)

1 large carrot, peeled and grated

1. In a food processor or blender, combine the peanut butter, soy sauce, rice vinegar, maple syrup, chili paste, and ginger. Blend into a paste, and then add enough water to create a slightly thinner sauce with the consistency of gravy. Set aside.

2. Fill a large pot with water and add the sea salt. Bring to a boil. Add the soba noodles, and cook according to the package directions. Once tender, drain the noodles and run under cold water to prevent clumping.

3. In a large bowl, toss the noodles with the sesame oil. Add the chicken, scallion greens, and carrot. Toss well. Add the sauce and stir to coat. Serve.

PER SERVING: Calories: 552, Protein: 39g, Cholesterol: 65mg, Sodium: 2,965mg, Total Carbohydrates: 57g, Fiber: 2g, Total Fat: 21g, Saturated Fat: 3g

"BUTTER" CHICKEN

DAIRY-FREE | GRAIN-FREE | GLUTEN-FREE | NUT-FREE | SOY-FREE |
KID-FRIENDLY | LOW-FODMAP

For a lot of people, eating out is one of the most difficult things to give up when undertaking this diet. Here, the Indian favorite Butter Chicken is reimagined without the onion (a heavily used component of most Indian cooking) or the ghee (clarified butter)—heart-healthy olive oil is used instead. You'll be surprised at how authentic this rich, creamy, "buttery" curry tastes. Serve over a bed of rice garnished with fresh cilantro.

SERVES 4

Prep time: 20 minutes, plus
  overnight marinating
Cook time: 35 minutes

---

1 pound boneless skinless chicken
  thighs, trimmed of fat and cut
  into 1-inch pieces
1½ teaspoons ground coriander
1 teaspoon sea salt
1 teaspoon cayenne pepper
½ teaspoon freshly cracked
  black pepper
½ teaspoon ground cumin
¼ teaspoon ground cinnamon
1 tablespoon plus 1 teaspoon fresh
  lemon juice
¼ cup extra virgin olive oil, divided
1 (15-ounce) can chopped
  tomatoes, drained
3 green cardamom pods
½ teaspoon ground mace
2-inch piece peeled fresh ginger,
  minced, divided
1 hot green chile pepper, seeded
  and minced
1 (15-ounce) can coconut milk
Fresh cilantro leaves, for garnish

1. In a large bowl, stir together the coriander, sea salt, cayenne pepper, black pepper, cumin, cinnamon, lemon juice, and 1 tablespoon of olive oil.

2. Add the chicken and toss until well coated. Cover and refrigerate overnight to marinate.

3. Preheat the oven to 400°F.

4. Arrange the chicken in a single layer on a baking sheet. Bake in the preheated oven for 15 minutes, until just barely cooked through. Remove from the oven and set aside.

5. In a saucepan over medium-high heat, heat 2 tablespoons of olive oil. Stir in the tomatoes, cardamom pods, mace, half the minced ginger, and the chile. Cook for 10 minutes until slightly thickened. Remove from the heat, and remove and discard the cardamom pods. Using a blender or an immersion blender, purée the mixture until smooth.

6. In a large saucepan over medium-high heat, heat the remaining tablespoon of olive oil. Add the remaining ginger and cook for about 45 seconds until fragrant.

7. Add the tomato purée and cooked chicken. Bring to a simmer. Stir in the coconut milk and reduce the heat to low. Cook for 5 to 7 minutes until heated through and the flavors meld. Serve immediately.

PER SERVING: Calories: 593, Protein: 36g, Cholesterol: 101mg, Sodium: 589mg, Total Carbohydrates: 11g, Fiber: 4g, Total Fat: 47g, Saturated Fat: 27g

Time-Saving Tip: Roast vegetables alongside your chicken. Roasted Brussels sprouts, asparagus, and cauliflower are all great accompaniments.

CHICKEN CHILI

GRAIN-FREE | GLUTEN-FREE | NUT-FREE | SOY-FREE | LOW-FODMAP

During Phase 1 you can still enjoy all the flavor of chili without the gut-irritating extras like onions, garlic, and beans. This dish is more stew-like, with zucchini, butternut squash, and Cheddar cheese. In Phase 2, this transitions into a white chili with the addition of beans (see Phase 2 Tip). Both versions are perfectly warming on cold days.

SERVES 4

Prep time: 15 minutes
Cook time: 50 minutes

1 teaspoon extra virgin olive oil
3 large boneless skinless chicken
    breasts, diced
1 red bell pepper, diced
1 small butternut squash, halved,
    seeded, peeled, and diced
4 cups Chicken Stock (page 100) or
    Vegetable Stock (page 99)
Juice of 1 lime
2 jalapeño peppers, diced
1 teaspoon ground cumin
1 teaspoon sweet paprika
½ teaspoon asafetida
¼ teaspoon cayenne pepper
2 small zucchini, diced
Sea salt
Freshly cracked black pepper
1 cup shredded Cheddar cheese

Phase 2 Tip: In step 1, add 2 (15.5-ounce) cans of reduced-sodium white kidney beans. In step 2 add 2 cups of frozen corn with the stock; omit the butternut squash.

1. In a large pot over medium-high heat, heat the olive oil. Add the chicken, red bell pepper, and butternut squash, and cook until the chicken is browned but not cooked through.

2. Stir in the chicken stock, lime juice, jalapeños, cumin, paprika, asafetida, and cayenne pepper. Bring to a boil, reduce the heat to low, and simmer for 30 to 40 minutes.

3. Stir in the zucchini and cook for 3 to 5 minutes just until the zucchini is tender.

4. Serve topped with Cheddar cheese.

PER SERVING: Calories: 415, Protein: 51g, Cholesterol: 127mg, Sodium: 1,205mg, Total Carbohydrates: 16g, Fiber: 4g, Total Fat: 17g, Saturated Fat: 7g

PESTO BAKED CHICKEN

GRAIN-FREE | GLUTEN-FREE | SOY-FREE | LOW-FODMAP

Packed with walnuts and Parmesan cheese, pesto is a protein-rich and nutrient-dense sauce that elevates any dish (try it with whitefish and salmon, too!). Serve this simple baked chicken alongside a nice green salad for a quick weeknight meal.

SERVES 4

Prep time: 15 minutes
Cook time: 35 minutes

For the pesto

1 cup tightly packed fresh basil leaves
⅓ cup unsalted walnuts
¼ cup grated Parmesan cheese
¼ cup extra virgin olive oil
Sea salt
Freshly cracked black pepper

For the chicken

4 boneless skinless chicken breasts
Sea salt
Freshly cracked black pepper
½ cup shredded mozzarella cheese

Time-Saving Tip: In the summer when basil is in season, double or triple the recipe to make large batches of pesto to freeze and have on hand throughout the year. Note, however, that to do this you must omit the Parmesan cheese, as it doesn't freeze well. When you are ready to use the pesto, just stir in the cheese, if desired.

To make the pesto

In a food processor, combine the basil, walnuts, Parmesan cheese, and olive oil. Process to a fine paste. Season to taste with sea salt and pepper.

To make the chicken

1. Preheat the oven to 400°F.

2. In a large bowl, place the chicken and season it to taste with sea salt and pepper.

3. Add the pesto and stir until the chicken is well coated.

4. Arrange the coated chicken in a single layer in a baking dish. Bake in the preheated oven for 20 to 30 minutes until the chicken is cooked through. Sprinkle evenly with the mozzarella cheese and bake for 3 to 5 more minutes, until the cheese is melted and bubbly.

PER SERVING: Calories: 628, Protein: 65g, Cholesterol: 179mg, Sodium: 730mg, Total Carbohydrates: 3g, Fiber: <1g, Total Fat: 40g, Saturated Fat: 11g

CHICKEN KEBABS

DAIRY-FREE | GRAIN-FREE | GLUTEN-FREE | NUT-FREE | SOY-FREE |
KID-FRIENDLY | LOW-FODMAP

Kebabs are classic dinner fare, perhaps because they are so simple to prepare and add some kid-friendly fun to the meal. If you can, cook these over a charcoal grill for a bit of natural smoked flavor. Otherwise, preheat your oven broiler while you thread the kebabs, and allow the meat to marinate for a full 30 minutes to really take on the mustard-maple flavor.

SERVES 4

Prep time: 15 minutes, plus
  30 minutes marinating
Cook time: 15 minutes

¼ cup pure maple syrup

¼ cup Dijon mustard

¼ cup water

½ teaspoon freshly cracked
    black pepper

1½ pounds boneless skinless chicken
    thighs and breasts, cut into small
    pieces, about 1½ inches wide

1 red bell pepper, cut into
    2-inch squares

1 small zucchini, sliced

1 small yellow squash, sliced

Ingredient Tip: If you are using wood skewers, soak them in water for at least 30 minutes before using to prevent scorching.

1. In a large bowl, whisk together the maple syrup, Dijon mustard, water, and pepper. Add the chicken and toss to coat well. Cover the bowl and refrigerate for 30 minutes.

2. Preheat the broiler to high.

3. Build your kebabs: thread alternating pieces of marinated chicken, bell pepper, zucchini, and yellow squash onto each skewer.

4. Place the kebabs on a baking sheet, and broil for about 8 minutes per side until the chicken is cooked through. Serve hot.

PER SERVING: Calories: 338, Protein: 51g, Cholesterol: 131mg, Sodium: 294mg, Total Carbohydrates: 18g, Fiber: 2g, Total Fat: 6g, Saturated Fat: 2g

CHICKEN PARMESAN

GLUTEN-FREE | NUT-FREE | SOY-FREE | KID-FRIENDLY | LOW-FODMAP

Chicken Parmesan is a classic dish that requires just a few tweaks to make it Phase 1 friendly. Be sure to whip up a batch of our Allium-Free Marinara Sauce (page 228), as many purchased brands contain onion and garlic, making them off-limits during Phase 1.

SERVES 4

Prep time: 15 minutes
Cook time: 45 minutes

---

1 teaspoon extra virgin olive oil

1¼ pounds boneless skinless chicken breasts, each cut lengthwise into 3 or 4 smaller cutlets (depending on their size)

2 cups Allium-Free Marinara Sauce (page 228) or purchased variety without onions and garlic

1 teaspoon dried basil

1 teaspoon dried oregano

1 (8-ounce) package fresh mozzarella cheese, cut into ½-inch cubes

¼ cup grated Parmesan cheese

1 cup gluten-free bread crumbs

Phase 2 Tip: You can save time by using a good-quality purchased marinara sauce instead of making it from scratch. Just be sure it contains no onions or garlic to be Phase 1 compliant.

1. Preheat the oven to 350°F.

2. Grease the bottom of a baking dish with the olive oil.

3. Lay the chicken cutlets in a single layer on the bottom of the baking dish.

4. Pour the marinara sauce over the chicken. Sprinkle with the basil and oregano, and top with the mozzarella and Parmesan cheeses. End with a layer of bread crumbs.

5. Bake in the preheated oven for 45 minutes until the top is well browned, and the chicken is cooked through.

PER SERVING: Calories: 601, Protein: 65g, Cholesterol: 162mg, Sodium: 1,372mg, Total Carbohydrates: 29g, Fiber: 3g, Total Fat: 25g, Saturated Fat: 11g

CHICKEN & RICE CASSEROLE

GLUTEN-FREE | NUT-FREE | SOY-FREE | KID-FRIENDLY | LOW-FODMAP

Casseroles are synonymous with comfort food, and this one delivers all the favorites—a creamy sauce, savory vegetables and poultry, and filling rice.

SERVES 6

Prep time: 15 minutes
Cook time: 1 hour

For the sauce

2 tablespoons butter
2 tablespoons rice flour
1 cup Vegetable Stock (page 99)
1 cup lactose-free milk or other nut milk
½ cup shredded Cheddar cheese
Sea salt
Freshly cracked black pepper

For the casserole

2 tablespoons butter, plus additional for greasing the baking dish
1 bunch fresh spinach, trimmed and roughly chopped
1 medium zucchini, diced
¼ cup chopped scallions (green part only)
4 cups cooked rice
2 cups cooked diced chicken (see Roast Chicken for Later, page 171)
1 cup Vegetable Stock (page 99)

To make the sauce

1. In a small saucepan over medium heat, melt the butter. Add the rice flour and cook, stirring constantly until a smooth paste forms.

2. While whisking, gradually pour in the vegetable stock and then the milk.

3. Add the Cheddar cheese and cook, whisking constantly until the cheese is melted. Season to taste with sea salt and pepper. Set aside.

To make the casserole

1. Preheat the oven to 350°F.

2. Grease an 8-by-8-inch baking dish with butter.

3. In a large skillet over medium heat, melt the 2 tablespoons of butter. Add the spinach, zucchini, and scallion greens. Cook for 2 minutes, stirring constantly until the spinach wilts and the zucchini just begins to soften. Turn off the heat.

4. To the same skillet, add the cooked rice and stir to combine.

5. Add the cooked chicken and stir to combine.

6. Whisk the vegetable stock into the sauce, then pour it over the rice mixture. Stir well.

7. Transfer the casserole to the prepared dish. Cover with aluminum foil, and bake in the preheated oven for 40 minutes until the casserole is bubbling. Uncover and bake for an additional 5 minutes until lightly browned on top.

PER SERVING: Calories: 457, Protein: 24g, Cholesterol: 70mg, Sodium: 588mg, Total Carbohydrates: 57g, Fiber: 2g, Total Fat: 14g, Saturated Fat: 8g

Phase 2 Tip: Add 2 cups of green beans or green peas to the casserole.

OVEN-BAKED CRISPY CHICKEN WINGS

DAIRY-FREE | NUT-FREE | KID-FRIENDLY | LOW-FODMAP

Oven-baked chicken wings are a sure crowd pleaser, even for the youngest set. These crispy wings won't disappoint and are free of sugars and other gut-aggravating ingredients. Serve with a quick salad or other side of your choice.

SERVES 4

Prep time: 10 minutes, plus
  30 minutes marinating
Cook time: 40 minutes to 1 hour

---

12 chicken wings
¼ cup soy sauce
½ teaspoon sea salt
**1 teaspoon freshly cracked
    black pepper**
½ teaspoon cayenne pepper
¼ cup extra virgin olive oil

Variation Tip: This recipe can be changed to suit your tastes. Replace the sea salt, black pepper, and cayenne pepper with any variation of your favorite spices, such as paprika, oregano, basil, or cumin.

1. With a sharp knife, split the wings by cutting between the drumette and middle section. Remove the wing tip in the same way by cutting between it and the middle section. Discard the wing tips or save them for making stock.

2. Place the chicken wings in a resealable bag and add the soy sauce; turn to coat well. Seal and refrigerate for 30 minutes.

3. Preheat the oven to 425°F.

4. Remove the wings from the marinade (discard the marinade) and place them in a large bowl. Season with the sea salt, black pepper, and cayenne pepper; stir until well coated.

5. Transfer the wings to a baking dish, drizzle with the olive oil, and toss so each wing is well coated.

6. Bake in the preheated oven for 30 to 40 minutes until well browned. Turn the wings over and bake for another 10 to 20 minutes until crispy. Serve hot.

PER SERVING: Calories: 549, Protein: 67g, Cholesterol: 202mg, Sodium: 1,328mg, Total Carbohydrates: 2g, Fiber: 0mg, Total Fat: 30g, Saturated Fat: 6g

STICKY CHICKEN WINGS

DAIRY-FREE | NUT-FREE

Sticky wings may be messy when dining out, but no one will see you licking your fingers when you make these at home. Because this recipe contains orange juice, you will have to wait until Phase 2 to dig in, but these tasty wings are worth the wait.

SERVES 4

Prep time: 10 minutes, plus
2 hours marinating
Cook time: 45 minutes

12 chicken wings
3 tablespoons fresh orange juice
2 tablespoons pure maple syrup
1 tablespoon sesame oil
1 tablespoon soy sauce
1 teaspoon Chinese five-
   spice powder
1 teaspoon grated orange zest
1-inch piece peeled fresh
   ginger, grated

Ingredient Tip: Chinese five-spice powder is a mixture of star anise, clove, cinnamon, Sichuan pepper, and fennel seeds. You can find it at Asian markets or well-stocked grocery stores.

1. With a sharp knife, split the wings by cutting between the drumette and middle section. Remove the wing tip in the same way by cutting between it and the middle section. Discard the wing tips or save them for making stock.

2. In a resealable bag, combine the orange juice, maple syrup, sesame oil, soy sauce, five-spice powder, orange zest, and ginger. Add the chicken, seal, and turn to mix and coat well. Refrigerate for at least 2 hours.

3. Preheat the oven to 425° F.

4. Line a baking sheet with parchment paper.

5. Remove the wings from the marinade, and arrange them in a single layer on the prepared sheet; reserve the marinade. Using a pastry brush, brush the wings with some of the reserved marinade. Bake in the preheated oven for 45 minutes, flipping once or twice, and brushing with marinade several times until they are cooked through and sticky. Serve hot.

PER SERVING: Calories: 496, Protein: 66g, Cholesterol: 202mg, Sodium: 422mg, Total Carbohydrates: 9g, Fiber: 0g, Total Fat: 20g, Saturated Fat: 5g

GREEN CURRY CHICKEN

DAIRY-FREE | GRAIN-FREE | GLUTEN-FREE | NUT-FREE | SOY-FREE | LOW-FODMAP

If you want to enjoy green curry, you are going to have to put in a little work to make the curry paste. Commercially available curry pastes are loaded with onions and garlic, which cannot be used during Phase 1 of the diet. Don't let that dissuade you from making green curry, though—the ingredients are readily available at well-stocked supermarkets and Asian grocers, and you'll be enjoying your warming curry before you know it!

SERVES 4

Prep time: 30 minutes
Cook time: 20 minutes

For the curry paste

2 stalks lemongrass
2 green Thai chiles
1 bunch scallions (green part only)
½ cup tightly packed fresh cilantro leaves and stems
½ cup tightly packed fresh Thai basil
1 tablespoon fresh lime juice
1 tablespoon pure maple syrup
½ teaspoon ground cumin
½ teaspoon ground coriander
½ teaspoon ground white pepper

For the curry

1 (15-ounce) can coconut milk
2 boneless skinless chicken breasts, thinly sliced
2 cups chopped Thai eggplant
1 tablespoon fish sauce
1 tablespoon pure maple syrup
1 tablespoon fresh lime juice

To make the curry paste

1. Prepare the lemongrass: Trim off the bottom of the lemongrass stalk and peel away the outer layers to reveal the pale lower stem. Cut the pale stem into thin pieces (discard everything else).

2. In a food processor, combine the chopped lemongrass, Thai chiles, scallion greens, cilantro, Thai basil, lime juice, maple syrup, cumin, coriander, and white pepper. Purée into a smooth paste. If necessary, add 1 or 2 tablespoons of water to loosen the mixture and aid processing.

To make the curry

1. Without shaking the can, open the coconut milk. Skim off about 2 tablespoons of the white solid coconut cream from the top (reserve the rest for the next step). Add the cream to a large skillet or wok over medium-high heat.

2. Add the curry paste and cook for about 30 seconds, stirring constantly until fragrant.

3. Add the chicken and cook for 3 to 4 minutes until browned.

4. Stir in the remaining coconut milk and eggplant, and bring to a boil. Reduce the heat to low and simmer for 10 to 15 minutes, stirring occasionally. When the chicken is cooked through and the eggplant is tender, turn off the heat and remove the pan from the burner.

5. Stir in the fish sauce, maple syrup, and lime juice. Taste and adjust seasonings, if desired. Serve hot.

PER SERVING: Calories: 514, Protein: 37g, Cholesterol: 101mg, Sodium: 470mg, Total Carbohydrates: 18g, Fiber: 5g, Total Fat: 34g, Saturated Fat: 25g

Ingredient Tip: Thai eggplant are green and circular. If you can't find them at an Asian market near you, substitute smaller purple Japanese or Chinese varieties (not the larger European variety).

TURKEY MEATBALLS

DAIRY-FREE | GLUTEN-FREE | NUT-FREE | SOY-FREE | KID-FRIENDLY | LOW-FODMAP

Let's face it: meatballs are fun and delicious. Here we provide a simple preparation you can dress up as you wish. Serve them on a salad, toss them with some gluten-free pasta and Parmesan cheese, drench them in Allium-Free Marinara Sauce (page 228), or simply pop them in your mouth one by one.

SERVES 4

Prep time: 15 minutes
Cook time: 25 minutes

——————

1 pound ground turkey
1 cup gluten-free bread crumbs
1 egg, beaten
1 teaspoon dried oregano
1 teaspoon dried sage
¾ teaspoon sea salt
½ teaspoon freshly cracked
    black pepper

Time-Saving Tip: If you find that the meat is too sticky when shaping it into balls, periodically wet your hands with water.

1. Preheat the oven to 350°F.

2. In a large bowl, break the turkey into smaller pieces. Add the bread crumbs, egg, oregano, sage, sea salt, and pepper. Using your hands, mix until well combined.

3. Pinch off tablespoon-size portions and shape into 1-inch balls.

4. Arrange the balls in a single layer on a rimmed baking sheet. Bake in the preheated oven for 20 to 25 minutes until browned and cooked through. Serve hot.

PER SERVING: Calories: 246, Protein: 36g, Cholesterol: 157mg, Sodium: 686mg, Total Carbohydrates: 20g, Fiber: 2g, Total Fat: 15g, Saturated Fat: 3g

TURKEY BREAST WITH HERBS

GRAIN-FREE | GLUTEN-FREE | NUT-FREE | SOY-FREE | KID-FRIENDLY | LOW-FODMAP

Turkey isn't just for Thanksgiving. Turkey breasts are available at the supermarket year-round and are just as easy to make during the week as they are for a classic Sunday supper. Try this easy oven-baked dish, which is loaded with herbs for big flavor. (Thaw a frozen turkey breast in the refrigerator for 2 days before using.)

SERVES 4

Prep time: 15 minutes
Cook time: 1 hour, 40 minutes,
  plus 10 minutes resting

---

1 (3- to 5-pound) bone-in skin-on
  turkey breast
3 tablespoons butter, melted
2 tablespoons chopped fresh
  rosemary leaves
1 tablespoon chopped fresh
  sage leaves
1 tablespoon chopped fresh
  thyme leaves
Zest of 1 lemon
Juice of 1 lemon
1 teaspoon sea salt
½ teaspoon freshly ground
  black pepper

Time-Saving Tip: Cut any leftovers into bite-size pieces and store in an airtight container. Use the turkey meat in the same way you would chicken for meals like Peanut-Ginger Chicken Soba Noodles (page 175) or Chicken & Rice Casserole (page 182).

1. Preheat the oven to 325°F.

2. Place the turkey breast on a roasting rack. In a small bowl, stir together the butter, rosemary, sage, thyme, lemon zest and juice, sea salt, and pepper. Using your hands, press this mixture firmly onto the top of the turkey breast so it sticks.

3. Arrange the turkey, breast-side down, on the roasting rack and cover loosely with aluminum foil. Roast in the preheated oven for 1 hour.

4. Remove the pan from the oven. Increase the oven temperature to 400°F. Using tongs, carefully turn the turkey breast-side up and return the pan to the oven, uncovered. Continue to roast for an additional 30 to 40 minutes until an instant-read thermometer registers 165°F at the thickest part of the breast.

5. Remove the pan from the oven and cover loosely with aluminum foil. Set aside for 10 minutes to rest. Carve and serve.

PER SERVING: Calories: 384, Protein: 49g, Cholesterol: 145mg, Sodium: 510mg, Total Carbohydrates: 14g, Fiber: 3g, Total Fat: 14g, Saturated Fat: 7g

SPICY BEEF CURRY

GLUTEN-FREE | NUT-FREE | SOY-FREE | LOW-FODMAP

Beef and other red meats should be enjoyed in moderation. When you want to indulge, this is a wonderfully seasoned dish that is friendly to the digestive system. Because you use an inexpensive cut of beef for this recipe, simmer the curry for a full hour to ensure the meat is tender.

SERVES 4

Prep time: 10 minutes
Cook time: 1 hour

¼ cup chopped scallions (green part only)
1½ teaspoons mustard seeds
1 dried red chile pepper
1-inch piece peeled fresh ginger, roughly chopped
1 tablespoon ghee
2 tablespoons curry powder
1 tablespoon ground turmeric
1 tablespoon white vinegar
1 tablespoon pure maple syrup
1 pound stewing beef
1 (15-ounce) can chopped tomatoes, with juice
½ cup Vegetable Stock (page 99) or water
1 cup unsweetened coconut milk

Ingredient Tip: Measure the spices before you begin cooking. If desired, place them in small individual bowls in the order in which they are needed so you can prevent scorching while looking for ingredients.

1. In a food processor, combine the scallion greens, mustard seeds, red chile pepper, and ginger and process to a smooth paste.

2. In a pot over medium-high heat, melt the ghee. Add the chile-ginger paste and cook for 15 to 20 seconds, stirring constantly.

3. Add the curry powder, turmeric, white vinegar, and maple syrup. Cook for 20 to 30 seconds, stirring constantly until fragrant.

4. Add the beef and tomatoes, stirring well to coat with the spices. Stir in the vegetable stock and bring to a boil. Reduce the heat to low, cover, and simmer for 30 minutes.

5. Stir in the coconut milk and cook for another 30 minutes more, uncovered, until the beef is tender (be careful not to let the curry boil or the milk may separate). Serve hot.

PER SERVING: Calories: 400, Protein: 29g, Cholesterol: 8mg, Sodium: 116mg, Total Carbohydrates:16g , Fiber: 5g, Total Fat: 26g, Saturated Fat: 15g

SLOW COOKER BEEF STEW

DAIRY-FREE | GRAIN-FREE | GLUTEN-FREE | NUT-FREE | SOY-FREE | KID-FRIENDLY

Using a slow cooker is one of the best ways to make beef stew because the meat benefits from low and slow cooking to tenderize it. If you don't have a slow cooker, the stove top works too, just keep the temperature on the lowest possible setting and check it regularly as you may need to add more water (you'll also need to adjust the cooking time to 3 hours). For some color on the plate and a bit of a textural contrast, serve with a side of steamed green beans or another green vegetable of your choice.

SERVES 6 TO 8

Prep time: 15 minutes

Cook time: 6 to 8 hours on low

---

2 pounds stewing beef

4 cups water

3 russet potatoes, peeled and cubed

3 carrots, chopped

1 cup chopped tomatoes, with juice

2 teaspoons dried oregano

2 teaspoons dried basil

1 teaspoon dried thyme

1 teaspoon sea salt

½ teaspoon freshly ground
    black pepper

Time-Saving Tip: To cut down on cleanup time, insert a slow cooker liner into your slow cooker before beginning.

In a slow cooker, combine the beef, water, potatoes, carrots, tomatoes, oregano, basil, thyme, sea salt, and pepper. Cover and cook for 6 to 8 hours on low. Serve hot.

PER SERVING: Calories: 419, Protein: 52g, Cholesterol: 80mg, Sodium: 514mg, Total Carbohydrates: 20g, Fiber: 4g, Total Fat: 14g, Saturated Fat: 3g

ROASTED PORK LOIN

DAIRY-FREE | GRAIN-FREE | GLUTEN-FREE | NUT-FREE | SOY-FREE |
KID-FRIENDLY | LOW-FODMAP

A warming combination of cumin, coriander, and turmeric (an anti-inflammatory), this simple dry rub transforms pork loin into a delectable meal. If you have a cast iron skillet, use it to make this recipe, as you can transfer it directly from the stove top to the oven. To complete the meal, serve this beautiful roast with a healthy side of Roasted Potatoes & Sweet Potatoes (page 126).

SERVES 4

Prep time: 10 minutes
Cook time: 40 minutes, plus
  5 minutes resting

2 teaspoons ground coriander
2 teaspoons ground cumin
1 teaspoon dried thyme
¾ teaspoon sea salt
½ teaspoon ground turmeric
1¼ pounds pork tenderloin
1 teaspoon coconut oil

Substitution Tip: If you don't have an oven-safe skillet, transfer the tenderloin from a skillet into a roasting dish before placing it in the oven.

1. Preheat the oven to 450°F.

2. In a small bowl, combine the coriander, cumin, thyme, sea salt, and turmeric. Rub the spice mix all over the tenderloin.

3. Heat an oven-safe skillet over medium-high heat. Melt the coconut oil. Add the pork and sear it on all sides, about 10 minutes total.

4. Transfer the skillet to the preheated oven and roast the tenderloin for 30 minutes, or until it reaches an internal temperature of 145°F. Remove the pan from the oven and let rest for 5 minutes. Slice and serve.

PER SERVING: Calories: 218, Protein: 37g, Cholesterol: 103mg, Sodium: 434mg, Total Carbohydrates: <1g, Fiber: 0g, Total Fat: 6g, Saturated Fat: 3g

FAMILY CABBAGE CASSEROLE

DAIRY-FREE | GLUTEN-FREE | NUT-FREE | SOY-FREE | LOW-FODMAP | KID-FRIENDLY

Making traditional cabbage rolls is a lot of work. This dish gives you the same flavor in a fraction of the time and makes a hearty one-dish meal that's good for the whole family. The casserole freezes well and leftovers are great for lunch the next day.

SERVES 6

Prep time: 10 minutes
Cook time: 1 hour

1 teaspoon extra virgin olive oil
1 pound extra-lean ground beef
2 teaspoons sea salt, divided
1 (28-ounce) can diced tomatoes, with juice
2 cups water
1 cup white rice
½ medium green cabbage, chopped
1 teaspoon dried oregano
¼ teaspoon freshly ground black pepper

Cooking Tip: When making this recipe in Phase 2, you can add extra flavor by frying ½ onion, chopped, along with the beef in step 2.

1. Preheat the oven to 350°F.

2. In a large skillet over medium heat, heat the olive oil. Add the ground beef and 1 teaspoon of sea salt. Cook for 7 to 10 minutes, stirring often until the ground beef is crumbled and browned. Drain off the liquid and transfer the beef to a large roasting pan.

3. Add the remaining teaspoon of sea salt, the tomatoes, water, rice, cabbage, oregano, and pepper. Stir well.

4. Cover and bake in the preheated oven for 30 minutes. Remove the pan from the oven and stir well. Re-cover and return to the oven for 30 to 35 minutes more until the rice is tender and the liquid has been absorbed. Serve hot.

PER SERVING: Calories: 290, Protein: 27g, Cholesterol: 68mg, Sodium: 688mg, Total Carbohydrates: 31g, Fiber: 3g, Total Fat: 6g, Saturated Fat: 2g

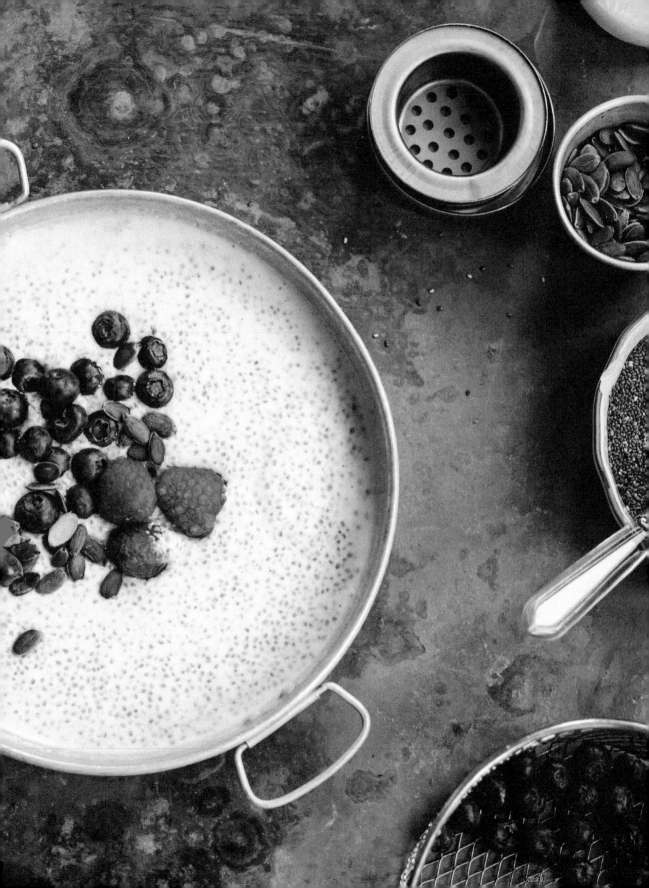

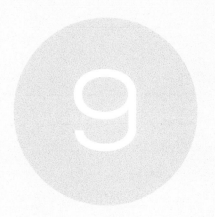

SNACKS & DESSERTS

As with everything, moderation is key. Choose 1 to 2 snacks per day to enjoy between meals and to keep you full and feeling great, and be sure to enjoy dessert once, or even twice, a week. When you make these healthier snack and dessert options, you don't have to leave your sweet tooth behind.

DRIED STRAWBERRIES

VEGAN | DAIRY-FREE | GRAIN-FREE | GLUTEN-FREE | NUT-FREE | SOY-FREE | KID-FRIENDLY

Drying strawberries during peak season allows you to enjoy their sweet flavor longer. Make these on a day you will be around the house, as they require a long drying time and watchful eye.

SERVES 4

Prep time: 10 minutes
Cook time: 3 to 4 hours,
  plus 1 hour cooling

1 pound strawberries, hulled; large berries cut into quarters, medium berries halved, and small berries left whole

Ingredient Tip: One cup of hulled and sliced strawberries is packed with as much vitamin C as 1 orange, and loaded with B vitamins, as well as vitamin A. They are in season in late spring and grow through August.

1. Preheat the oven to 200°F.

2. Line a baking sheet with parchment paper.

3. Arrange the strawberries cut-side up in a single layer on the prepared baking sheet.

4. Bake in the preheated oven for 3 to 4 hours, rotating the sheet every 45 minutes or so to promote even cooking. When done, the strawberries will not be crisp, but will be shrunken and pliable, with no excess moisture.

5. Remove from the oven and let cool for 1 hour. If the strawberries do not begin to crisp after cooling for 15 minutes, return them to the oven and bake for 20 minutes more and try again.

PER SERVING: Calories: 36, Protein: <1g, Cholesterol: 0mg, Sodium: 1mg, Total Carbohydrates: 9g, Fiber: 2g, Total Fat: <1g, Saturated Fat: 0g

DRIED BANANAS

VEGAN | DAIRY-FREE | GRAIN-FREE | GLUTEN-FREE | NUT-FREE |

SOY-FREE | KID-FRIENDLY | LOW-FODMAP

Purchased dried banana chips are delicious, but often loaded with sugar and/or high fructose corn syrup. Fortunately, they are fairly easy to make at home. Be sure to use just-ripe bananas, when the flesh is still somewhat firm, so you can cut thin slices.

SERVES 4

Prep time: 10 minutes
Cook time: 2 to 3 hours,
   plus 1 hour cooling

**2 to 3 large bananas, cut into
   ⅛-inch rounds**

2 tablespoons fresh lemon juice

Variation Tip: Dried banana chips taste great with the concentrated natural sugars and flavor of banana, but if you would like a little extra pizzazz, add a sprinkle of cinnamon to each piece.

1. Preheat the oven to 225°F.

2. Line a baking sheet with parchment paper.

3. Arrange the banana slices in a single layer on the prepared baking sheet. Using a pastry brush, coat both sides of the banana slices with lemon juice.

4. Bake in the preheated oven for 2 to 3 hours, checking after 1 hour, and then again at 20-minute intervals until done. They are ready when shrunken and dehydrated looking.

5. Remove from the oven and let cool on the baking sheet for 1 hour. If they do not begin to crisp after cooling for 10 minutes, return to the oven and bake for 20 minutes more and try again.

PER SERVING: Calories: 81, Protein: 1g, Cholesterol: 0mg, Sodium: 2mg, Total Carbohydrates: 20g, Fiber: 2g, Total Fat: <1g, Saturated Fat: 0g

SUPER NUTTY TRAIL MIX

VEGAN | GRAIN-FREE | GLUTEN-FREE | SOY-FREE | LOW-FODMAP

Many of the ingredients in classic trail mix are a no-go when repairing the gut. Laden with dried fruits and candies, they can do more harm than good. However, you can easily make your own for a portable snack on the go. Stored in an airtight container, it will stay fresh for up to 1 week.

MAKES 3¾ CUPS

Prep time: 5 minutes
Cook time: 15 minutes

---

1 cup chopped unsalted walnuts
1 cup raw unsalted sunflower seeds
1 cup raw unsalted pumpkin seeds
½ cup dark chocolate chips
¼ cup shredded
    unsweetened coconut

Variation Tip: Oats, peanuts, and macadamia nuts can all be substituted for the nuts and seeds in this recipe in equal proportions.

1. Preheat the oven to 350°F.

2. Arrange the walnuts, sunflower seeds, and pumpkin seeds in an even layer on a baking sheet. Bake for 10 to 15 minutes, stirring occasionally to prevent scorching until golden brown and fragrant.

3. Remove the baking sheet from the oven and set aside to cool completely.

4. Add the chocolate chips and coconut and mix well. Store in an airtight container.

PER SERVING: (Per cup): Calories: 570, Protein: 21g, Cholesterol: 0mg, Sodium: 9mg, Total Carbohydrates: 24g, Fiber: 5g, Total Fat: 49g, Saturated Fat: 9g

CURRIED WALNUTS

VEGETARIAN | GRAIN-FREE | GLUTEN-FREE | SOY-FREE | LOW-FODMAP

Nuts are a quick snack on their own, but adding curry powder makes them even better. You can use any nuts you prefer, but here we use heart-healthy walnuts. Note that this recipe includes salt; if you are using salted nuts, there's no need to add any extra.

MAKES 2 CUPS

Prep time: 5 minutes
Cook time: 45 minutes

---

1 tablespoons butter, melted
2 tablespoons curry powder
½ teaspoon sea salt
2 cups unsalted walnuts

Time-Saving Tip: These nuts can be made up to 3 weeks in advance, so make a double or triple batch to have on hand when hunger hits.

1. Preheat the oven to 250°F.

2. In a large bowl, mix the melted butter, curry powder, and sea salt. Add the walnuts and toss until well coated.

3. Spread the seasoned nuts in a single layer on a baking sheet.

4. Bake for 45 minutes, stirring every 10 to 15 minutes until dried. Let cool completely on the baking sheet, and then transfer to an airtight container.

PER SERVING: (Per half-cup): Calories: 422, Protein: 16g, Cholesterol: 8mg, Sodium: 257mg, Total Carbohydrates: 8g, Fiber: 5g, Total Fat: 40g, Saturated Fat: 4g

MAPLE-CAYENNE ROASTED ALMONDS

VEGAN | SOY-FREE | GRAIN-FREE | LOW-FODMAP

Spicy and sweet, these almonds are made for snacking. Cinnamon, a warming spice, and cayenne pepper are both great digestive aids. Make these ahead of time, and store them for up to 2 weeks.

MAKES 2 CUPS

Prep time: 5 minutes
Cook time: 20 minutes

⅓ cup pure maple syrup
1 tablespoon ground cinnamon
1 teaspoon cayenne pepper
2 cups raw unsalted almonds
Sea salt

Ingredient Tip: When shopping for almonds, choose organic whenever possible. Organic almonds are flash pasteurized, while commercial varieties are sprayed with a fumigant, propylene oxide, which is a suspected carcinogen. Because almonds can absorb odors of surrounding foods, it is important to store them in an airtight container.

1. Preheat the oven to 325°F.

2. Line a baking sheet with parchment paper.

3. In a medium bowl, whisk together the maple syrup, cinnamon, and cayenne pepper. Add the almonds and stir to coat well. Spread the nuts in a single layer on the prepared baking sheet and sprinkle lightly with sea salt.

4. Bake in the preheated oven for 10 minutes. Remove from the oven and stir well. Return the baking sheet to the oven and bake for 10 minutes more.

5. Remove from the oven and let cool for 20 minutes before serving. Store cooled nuts in an airtight container.

PER SERVING: (per half cup): Calories: 348, Protein: 10g, Cholesterol: 0mg, Sodium: 62mg, Total Carbohydrates: 29g, Fiber: 7g, Total Fat: 24g, Saturated Fat: 2g

ROASTED CHICKPEAS

VEGAN | DAIRY-FREE | GRAIN-FREE | GLUTEN-FREE | NUT-FREE | SOY-FREE

Until you try oven-roasted chickpeas, you probably won't believe how wonderful they really are. By baking them twice, the chickpeas become perfectly crunchy. With the addition of a few spices, they become addictively savory, too.

MAKES 3 CUPS

Prep time: 5 minutes
Cook time: 1 hour, plus
  20 minutes resting

---

2 (15-ounce) cans low-sodium
  chickpeas, rinsed and drained
2 tablespoons extra virgin olive oil
1 teaspoon ground cumin
1 teaspoon chili powder
½ teaspoon sea salt

*Phase 2 Tip: If you can tolerate
it, add 1 minced garlic clove to
the chickpeas.*

1. Preheat the oven to 400°F.

2. Spread the chickpeas over a paper towel and then cover with a second paper towel. Pat dry.

3. In a large bowl, stir together the chickpeas, olive oil, cumin, chili powder, and sea salt. Spread evenly over a baking sheet.

4. Bake in the preheated oven for 30 minutes. Remove from the oven (keep the oven on) and let the chickpeas cool for 15 to 20 minutes, or until cooled completely. Return the baking sheet to the oven and bake for 30 minutes more. Remove from the oven, let cool, and serve.

PER SERVING: (per half cup): Calories: 599, Protein: 28g, Cholesterol: 0mg, Sodium: 195mg, Total Carbohydrates: 86g, Fiber: 25g, Total Fat: 13g, Saturated Fat: 2g

POPPED CORN THREE WAYS

VEGETARIAN | NUT-FREE | SOY-FREE | LOW-FODMAP

Making popcorn on the stove can be tricky, but with this recipe, you'll quickly become a pro. The secret is to bring all the kernels to roughly the same temperature before popping begins, to ensure you pop as many kernels as possible and prevent scorching. Once your popcorn is ready, choose the traditional buttered variety, or add nori or nutritional yeast seasonings.

MAKES 2 QUARTS
Prep time: 5 minutes
Cook time: 10 minutes

For the popped corn
2 tablespoons coconut oil
⅓ cup popcorn kernels

For traditional buttered popped corn
1 tablespoon butter
Sea salt

For nori-seasoned popped corn
2 sheets nori, torn into small pieces
1 tablespoon togarashi seasoning

For nutritional yeast-seasoned popped corn
3 tablespoons nutritional yeast

To make the popped corn

1. In a large pot with a lid over medium-high heat, melt the coconut oil. Add 3 popcorn kernels and cover the pan.

2. When the kernels pop, add the remaining popcorn, cover the pot with the lid, and shake well. Remove the pot from the heat for 30 seconds, shaking a couple times to distribute the heat evenly.

3. Return the pot to the heat, shaking regularly over the burner. Once the popcorn begins popping, continue shaking the pan. When the popcorn slows to popping just every few seconds, remove from the heat and transfer the popcorn to a large bowl.

To make traditional buttered popped corn
Add the butter to the hot pot and swirl it several times to melt the butter. Pour the melted butter over the popcorn and season to taste with sea salt. ▶

Ingredient Tip: Togarashi seasoning is a seven-spice chili seasoning from Japan. It typically contains ground chile peppers, orange peel, sesame seeds, poppy seeds, hemp seeds, ginger, and nori. It can be found at any Asian market or well-stocked grocery store.

To make nori-seasoned popped corn

1. In a food processor fitted with the metal blade, place the nori. Add the togarashi seasoning. Pulse to a powder.

2. Toss the seasoning with the buttered popped corn and serve.

To make the nutritional yeast-seasoned popped corn

Toss the buttered popped corn with the nutritional yeast and serve.

PER SERVING: Calories: 107, Protein: <1g, Cholesterol: 8mg, Sodium: 138mg, Total Carbohydrates: 5g, Fiber: <1g, Total Fat: 10g, Saturated Fat: 8g

JERUSALEM ARTICHOKE CHIPS

VEGAN | DAIRY-FREE | GRAIN-FREE | GLUTEN-FREE | NUT-FREE | SOY-FREE

When that potato chip craving hits, satisfy the urge with these Jerusalem artichoke chips. Simply flavored, this classic recipe has great taste and big crunch. Only make one batch of these at a time, as they are best enjoyed the same day they are made.

MAKES 4 SERVINGS

Prep time: 15 minutes, plus
  30 minutes resting
Cook time: 30 minutes

1 pound Jerusalem artichokes,
  cleaned and ends trimmed off
¾ teaspoon sea salt, divided
1 tablespoon extra virgin olive oil

Variation Tip: Paprika, rosemary, and thyme all pair well with the subtle flavor of Jerusalem artichoke chips. Play around with both fresh and dried herbs to find the flavor combinations that you enjoy most.

1. Using a mandoline, slice the artichokes into ⅛-inch rounds and transfer to a large bowl. Toss the pieces with ½ teaspoon sea salt and set aside for 30 minutes to rest.

2. Preheat the oven to 350°F.

3. Line a large baking sheet with parchment paper.

4. Place the artichoke slices in the center of a clean paper towel or kitchen towel and press out as much liquid as you can. Arrange the slices in a single layer on the prepared sheet.

5. Using a pastry brush, coat both sides of the slices with the olive oil. Season with the remaining ¼ teaspoon of sea salt.

6. Bake in the preheated oven for 30 minutes until crisp and golden brown.

PER SERVING: Calories: 30, Protein: 4g, Cholesterol: 0mg, Sodium: 458mg, Total Carbohydrates: 12g, Fiber: 6g, Total Fat: 4, Saturated Fat: <1g

KALE CHIPS

VEGAN | DAIRY-FREE | GRAIN-FREE | GLUTEN-FREE | NUT-FREE | SOY-FREE | LOW-FODMAP

When done well, kale chips are an easy stand-in for fried potato chips. The trick is to dry the leaves well after washing, remove all the stems, tear the leaves into a uniform size, and bake them on low so they cook slowly to perfection.

MAKES 4 SERVINGS

Prep time: 5 minutes
Cook time: 30 minutes

---

1 bunch kale, stems removed and
     leaves torn into uniform pieces
1½ teaspoons extra virgin olive oil
1 tablespoon nutritional yeast
¼ teaspoon sea salt
⅛ teaspoon cayenne pepper

Variation Tip: You can also make chips from collard greens in the same way. Be sure to remove all large woody stems. Follow the recipe, but add an additional 10 to 15 minutes to the cooking time, as needed.

1. Preheat the oven to 300°F.

2. Line a baking sheet with parchment paper.

3. In a large bowl, combine the kale leaves and olive oil. Using clean hands, massage the oil into the kale until it is well coated. Sprinkle with the nutritional yeast, sea salt, and cayenne pepper. Stir to combine.

4. Spread the kale in a single layer on the prepared sheet. Bake in the preheated oven for 10 minutes, rotate the pan, and continue baking for 15 minutes more. Remove from the oven and let cool for 5 minutes before serving.

PER SERVING: Calories: 57, Protein: 3g, Cholesterol: 0mg, Sodium: 148mg, Total Carbohydrates: 8g, Fiber: 2g, Total Fat: 2g, Saturated Fat: 0g

ZUCCHINI CHIPS

VEGETARIAN | GRAIN-FREE | GLUTEN-FREE | SOY-FREE | LOW-FODMAP

Zucchini is inexpensive, and if you are lucky enough to have some gardening space, grows abundantly when warm weather hits. Here's a different way to enjoy it: cover slices in a tasty Parmesan and gluten-free bread crumb coating and bake it to a crisp.

MAKES 4 CUPS

Prep time: 10 minutes
Cook time: 30 minutes

Cooking spray

¼ cup gluten-free bread crumbs

¼ cup grated Parmesan cheese

¼ teaspoon sea salt

¼ teaspoon freshly ground
    black pepper

2 tablespoons unsweetened coconut
    milk, almond milk, or nut milk

2 small zucchini, cut into
    ¼-inch rounds

Variation Tip: Make these chips with yellow squash when available.

1. Preheat the oven to 425°F.

2. Spray an ovenproof wire rack with nonstick cooking spray and place on a large baking sheet.

3. Set up a breading station: In a small bowl, combine the bread crumbs, Parmesan cheese, sea salt, and pepper and stir well. In another small bowl, add the milk.

4. Dip the zucchini slices in the milk, then roll them in the seasoned bread crumbs, pressing the mixture onto the zucchini's surface to stick.

5. Arrange the zucchini slices in a single layer on the rack, and bake for 30 minutes, until browned and crisp. Serve hot.

PER SERVING: Calories: 83, Protein: 5g, Cholesterol: 5mg, Sodium: 243mg, Total Carbohydrates: 9g, Fiber: 2g, Total Fat: 4g, Saturated Fat: 3g

DEVILED EGGS

VEGETARIAN | GRAIN-FREE | NUT-FREE | SOY-FREE | LOW-FODMAP

Deviled eggs are easy to prepare and make a wonderful snack. Once prepared, the eggs can be refrigerated for up to 3 days.

SERVES 4

Prep time: 15 minutes

6 hardboiled eggs, peeled and
    halved lengthwise
¼ cup mayonnaise
Pinch cayenne pepper
Sea salt
Freshly ground black pepper
Paprika, for garnish
Chopped fresh chives, for garnish

Variation Tip: For a super creamy texture, reduce the amount of mayonnaise to 2 tablespoons and add 1 mashed avocado to the egg yolks.

1. Into a small mixing bowl, scoop the egg yolks. Set the egg whites aside.

2. Using a fork, mash the yolks. Stir in the mayonnaise and the cayenne pepper. Season to taste with sea salt and pepper. Stir to combine.

3. Using a teaspoon, fill the egg whites with the yolk mixture. Garnish with paprika and chives.

PER SERVING: Calories: 152, Protein: 8g, Cholesterol: 249mg, Sodium: 314mg, Total Carbohydrates: 4g, Fiber: 0g, Total Fat: 12g, Saturated Fat: 3g

POMEGRANATE-BERRY GUMMIES

DAIRY-FREE | GRAIN-FREE | NUT-FREE | SOY-FREE | KID-FRIENDLY

Gelatin, the solidifying ingredient in gummy snacks, is great for gut health, but all the fillers and sweeteners in commercial gummy brands make them a not-so-great choice for snacking. However, this simple recipe will have you back in gummy business for good. Because this snack uses fruit juice, which is high in fructose, it is best to make these in Phase 2. You will need three small silicone molds for this recipe, or you can use a baking dish lined with plastic wrap or greased with mild-tasting oil, such as vegetable oil or refined coconut oil.

MAKES 25 GUMMIES

Prep time: 5 minutes
Cook time: 10 minutes, plus
  2 to 3 hours chilling and 5 to
  10 minutes freezing

1½ cups pomegranate juice
2 tablespoons pure maple
    syrup, optional
1½ cups frozen mixed berries
    (blueberries, raspberries,
    blackberries), puréed
6 tablespoons gelatin powder

Ingredient Tip: Pomegranates are high in pantothenic acid, also known as vitamin B$_5$, an important vitamin in the body's assimilation of carbohydrates, fats, and protein. They also contain a tannin, punicalagin, which is helpful in protecting the body from cancer.

1. In a small saucepan over low heat, heat the pomegranate juice until just starting to steam, but not simmering yet. Stir in the maple syrup (if using) and the mixed berries.

2. Whisking constantly, pour the gelatin in a steady stream into the mixture. Take care to mix the gelatin until smooth.

3. Carefully pour the mixture into silicone molds and refrigerate for 2 to 3 hours to set. To remove the gummies from the molds, freeze for 5 to 10 minutes to harden, and then pop them out. Refrigerate in an airtight container for up to 10 days.

PER SERVING: (per gummy) Calories: 24, Protein: 2g, Cholesterol: 0mg, Sodium: 4mg, Total Carbohydrates: 5g, Fiber: 0mg, Total Fat: 0g, Saturated Fat: 0g

5-MINUTE COCONUT CHIA PUDDING

VEGAN | GRAIN-FREE | GLUTEN-FREE | SOY-FREE | LOW-FODMAP

This chia seed and coconut pudding comes together in minutes—about five is all you need! Top it with your favorite fresh fruit for a sweet and creamy treat.

MAKES 4 CUPS

Prep time: 5 minutes,
  plus 2 hours chilling

½ cup chia seeds, divided

4 cups full-fat unsweetened coconut milk, almond milk, or soy milk, divided

2 tablespoons pure maple syrup, divided

Nuts, seeds, berries, or fruits of choice, for serving

Variation Tip: For a richer pudding, substitute an equal amount of coconut cream for the milk.

1. Have ready 4 jars or cups with lids (large enough to hold 1 cup of milk each). To each jar, add 2 tablespoons of chia seeds, 1 cup of milk, and 1½ teaspoons of maple syrup.

2. Cover the jars with the lids and shake each jar vigorously to combine well. Refrigerate for 2 hours or as long as overnight. Serve topped with nuts, seeds, berries, or other fruits. (The puddings will keep refrigerated in airtight containers for up to 3 days.)

PER SERVING: Calories: 700, Protein: 10g, Cholesterol: 0mg, Sodium: 42mg, Total Carbohydrates: 32g, Fiber: 15g, Total Fat: 66g, Saturated Fat: 51g

CHOCOLATE CHIA PUDDING

VEGAN | GRAIN-FREE | GLUTEN-FREE | SOY-FREE | LOW-FODMAP

Although this chocolatey chia pudding tastes decadent, it's actually good for you. Chia seeds are loaded with fiber and protein. They also boast a high level of antioxidants, which help fight free radicals, and have high levels of omega-3 fatty acids, calcium, and magnesium. Grinding the chia seeds yields a uniform texture to the finished pudding. If you don't mind a little texture, leave them whole.

MAKES 4 CUPS

Prep time: 5 minutes,
  plus 2 hours chilling

---

4 teaspoons unsweetened cocoa
  powder, divided

2 tablespoons pure maple
  syrup, divided

½ cup chia seeds, ground, divided

4 cups full-fat unsweetened coconut
  milk, almond milk, or soy
  milk, divided

Ingredient Tip: When using ground chia seeds, they should be ground just before using. Use a clean spice grinder or coffee grinder to grind chia seeds to a fine powder.

1. Have ready 4 cups or jars with lids (large enough to hold 1 cup of milk each). To each jar, add 1 teaspoon of cocoa powder, 1½ teaspoons of maple syrup, and 2 tablespoons of chia seeds and stir well. Add 1 cup of coconut milk to each jar.

2. Cover the jars with the lids and shake vigorously to combine well. Refrigerate for at least 2 hours or as long as overnight. Serve. (The puddings will keep refrigerated in airtight containers for up to 3 days.)

PER SERVING: Calories: 704, Protein: 10g, Cholesterol: 0mg, Sodium: 69mg, Total Carbohydrates: 33g, Fiber: 15g, Total Fat: 66g, Saturated Fat: 51g

DARK CHOCOLATE MELTS

VEGAN | GRAIN-FREE | GLUTEN-FREE | SOY-FREE | KID-FRIENDLY | LOW-FODMAP

These tiny little chocolate bites are hugely satisfying and loaded with omega-3 fatty acids, fiber, and antioxidants. Look for a chocolate with a high percentage (at least 85 percent) cacao for the healthiest choice, and be sure to buy a bar, not chips that use additives to prevent melting.

MAKES 20 PIECES

Prep time: 10 minutes, plus 2 to
  3 hours chilling

---

1 tablespoon chopped
  unsalted walnuts
1 tablespoon chopped
  unsalted almonds
1 tablespoon chia seeds
1 tablespoon dried unsweetened
  coconut flakes
1 (8-ounce) bar extra-dark
  (85 percent cacao) chocolate,
  chopped into small pieces

*Phase 2 Tip: Add dried fruits such as
figs, goji berries, apricots, and dates.*

1. Line a baking sheet with wax paper or parchment paper.

2. In a small bowl, mix the walnuts, almonds, chia seeds, and coconut. Set aside.

3. Place the chocolate in a microwave-safe glass container and microwave for 60 seconds on high. Stir the chocolate, then microwave for 30 seconds more, or until the chocolate is completely melted.

4. Using a small spoon, drop small chocolate rounds (about the size of a quarter) onto the prepared sheet. Sprinkle with the coconut-nut mixture.

5. Refrigerator for 2 to 3 hours, until fully set.

PER SERVING: (per piece) Calories: 68, Protein: 1g, Cholesterol: 3mg, Sodium: 9mg, Total Carbohydrates: 7g, Fiber: <1g, Total Fat: 4g, Saturated Fat: 3g

FLOURLESS BROWNIES

VEGETARIAN | GRAIN-FREE | GLUTEN-FREE | SOY-FREE | KID-FRIENDLY

Living a low-gluten lifestyle doesn't have to be boring when it comes to dessert. Almond meal replaces the flour in these rich, chocolatey brownies. Use a good-quality unsweetened cocoa powder for the best flavor.

MAKES 12 BROWNIES

Prep time: 15 minutes
Cook time: 30 minutes

Cooking spray
¾ cup almond meal
¼ cup unsweetened cocoa powder
1 teaspoon baking powder
¼ teaspoon sea salt
½ cup butter
½ cup granulated sugar
3 large eggs
1 teaspoon pure vanilla extract
¼ cup dark chocolate chips

Variation Tip: Add about ¾ cup of walnuts to the brownie mix for a heartier brownie with a bit of crunch.

1. Preheat the oven to 350°F.

2. Spray an 8-by-8-inch baking pan with nonstick cooking spray.

3. In a large bowl, mix the almond meal, cocoa powder, baking powder, and sea salt. Set aside.

4. In a small saucepan over medium heat, melt the butter. Add the sugar and stir to combine. Turn off the heat.

5. In a small bowl, whisk together the eggs and vanilla. Fold in the butter-sugar mixture. Add the egg mixture all at once to the almond mixture and stir well. Fold in the dark chocolate chips.

6. Pour the batter into the prepared baking dish. Bake for 30 minutes, or until a dry toothpick inserted into the center comes out fairly clean (a little bit of gooeyness is okay). Let cool in the pan. Cut into 12 even squares. Serve immediately or store in an airtight container for up to 5 days.

PER SERVING: (per brownie) Calories: 169, Protein: 3g, Cholesterol: 67mg, Sodium: 112mg, Total Carbohydrates: 13g, Fiber: 1g, Total Fat: 13g, Saturated Fat: 6g

CHOCOLATE-PEANUT BUTTER COOKIES

VEGETARIAN | GRAIN-FREE | GLUTEN-FREE | SOY-FREE | KID-FRIENDLY | LOW-FODMAP

Using banana in baked goods is a great way to get around added sugar—an overripe banana is loaded with natural sugar. And, because these chocolate-peanut butter cookies contain no refined sugar, they're a great choice for this diet. You'll find it hard to eat just one.

MAKES 12 COOKIES

Prep time: 15 minutes
Cook time: 15 minutes

---

2 dark and very ripe bananas
6 tablespoons coconut flour
2 tablespoons peanut butter
2 tablespoons unsweetened
    cocoa powder
½ teaspoon baking powder
⅛ teaspoon sea salt
½ cup unsweetened lactose-free milk
    or nut milk
¼ cup dark chocolate chips

Time-Saving Tip: There is no reason to make cookies every time your bananas start looking a little dark. Instead, peel the bananas and pop them in a freezer-safe bag or container and freeze them until ready to use.

1. Preheat the oven to 350°F.

2. Line a baking sheet with parchment paper.

3. In a food processor fitted with the metal blade, combine the bananas, coconut flour, peanut butter, cocoa powder, baking powder, sea salt, and milk. Process until uniform in texture. Remove the blade.

4. Using your hands, scoop out about 1 tablespoon of dough and roll it into a ball. Place it on the prepared baking sheet and, using the palm of your hand, press down gently to flatten. Repeat, spacing the cookies at least 2 inches apart, until all of the dough is used. Sprinkle the dough rounds with the chocolate chips.

5. Bake in the preheated oven for 15 minutes until lightly browned. Remove from the oven and let cool on the baking sheet. Store in an airtight container for up to 5 days.

PER SERVING: (per cookie) Calories: 61, Protein: 2g, Cholesterol: 1mg, Sodium: 38mg, Total Carbohydrates: 8g, Fiber: 1g, Total Fat: 3g, Saturated Fat: 2g

OATMEAL CHOCOLATE-CHIP COOKIES

VEGETARIAN | NUT-FREE | SOY-FREE | KID-FRIENDLY | LOW-FODMAP

Oatmeal cookies have never tasted so good—or been so easy to make. Sweetened with ripe bananas to minimize the need for refined sugars, and packed with fiber-rich oatmeal to keep you satisfied longer, you can enjoy these as a healthier, delicious dessert option. If you have kids, get them to lend you a hand with this recipe.

MAKES 12 COOKIES

Prep time: 5 minutes, plus
  5 minutes resting
Cook time: 20 minutes

---

2 very ripe bananas
1 cup quick-cooking rolled oats
¼ cup semi-sweet chocolate chips
1 teaspoon pure vanilla extract
½ teaspoon ground cinnamon

Phase 2 Tip: Add up to ⅓ cup dried fruits, such as goji berries, cranberries, and golden raisins, to the cookies, if desired.

1. Preheat the oven to 350°F.

2. Line a baking sheet with parchment paper.

3. In a medium bowl, mash the bananas until liquid-like. Stir in the oats, chocolate chips, vanilla, and cinnamon. Let the mixture stand for 5 minutes.

4. Using a tablespoon, drop mounds of dough onto the prepared sheet, spacing at least 2 inches apart, and press down gently to flatten.

5. Bake in the preheated oven for 20 minutes until golden brown. Let cool completely on the sheet. Store in an airtight container.

PER SERVING: (per cookie) Calories: 57, Protein: 1g, Cholesterol: 1mg, Sodium: 3mg, Total Carbohydrates: 11g, Fiber: 1g, Total Fat: 1g, Saturated Fat: <1g

PEANUT BUTTER-LENTIL BARS

VEGETARIAN | DAIRY-FREE | KID-FRIENDLY

These tasty bars are so good the kids will never know they're full of fiber! Pack these in school or work lunches or enjoy them as a quick breakfast-on-the-go.

SERVES 6

Prep time: 20 minutes
Bake time: 25 minutes

Cooking spray
½ cup dried red lentils, rinsed and drained
1¼ cups water, divided
1 cup spelt flour
½ cup natural peanut butter
⅓ cup pure maple syrup
1 egg
1 tablespoon pure vanilla extract
1 teaspoon baking powder
½ teaspoon baking soda
½ teaspoon sea salt
¼ cup carob chips

Cooking Tip: Make this bar gluten-free by substituting gluten-free all-purpose flour for the spelt flour (the texture may differ slightly).

1. Preheat the oven to 350°F.

2. Spray a 9-by-9-inch baking pan with nonstick cooking spray and set aside.

3. In a large saucepan over medium heat, combine the lentils and 1 cup of water. Cook for about 15 minutes, stirring often until the liquid is absorbed. Remove from the heat and let cool for 10 minutes.

4. In a blender, combine the cooked lentils, spelt flour, peanut butter, maple syrup, egg, vanilla, baking powder, baking soda, sea salt, and the remaining ¼ cup of water. Blend on medium until smooth.

5. Using a spatula, scrape the mixture into the prepared pan. Sprinkle the carob chips evenly over the top.

6. Bake in the preheated oven for 20 to 25 minutes. Remove from the oven and let cool in the pan. Slice into squares. Store in an airtight container at room temperature for up to 5 days.

PER SERVING: Calories: 339, Protein: 14g, Cholesterol: 27mg, Sodium: 379mg, Total Carbohydrates: 43g, Fiber: 9g, Total Fat: 14g, Saturated Fat: 4g

CANTALOUPE-MAPLE GRANITA

VEGAN | DAIRY-FREE | GRAIN-FREE | GLUTEN-FREE | NUT-FREE | SOY-FREE |
KID-FRIENDLY | LOW-FODMAP

On a hot day, there's nothing better than a cold, refreshing granita—a semi-frozen dessert that originated in Italy. Cantaloupe is a low-fructose fruit, making it suitable for Phase 1.

SERVES 4

Prep time: 10 minutes, plus
  2 to 3 hours freezing

1 large cantaloupe, halved, seeded,
    peeled, and cut into chunks
3 tablespoons pure maple syrup
Fresh mint leaves, for garnish

Phase 2 Tip: Make a granita with other types of fruits using this same method. Strawberries, watermelon, honeydew melon, and peaches all make great granitas.

1. In a blender, combine the cantaloupe and maple syrup and process until smooth. Pour the mixture into a 9-by-13-inch baking dish, and freeze for 2 to 3 hours.

2. Using the tines of a fork, scrape and break up the frozen mixture into granules.

3. Divide evenly among 4 small cups. Garnish with mint leaves and serve.

PER SERVING: Calories: 92 , Protein: 1g, Cholesterol: 0mg, Sodium: 26mg, Total Carbohydrates: 23g, Fiber: 1g, Total Fat: <1g, Saturated Fat: 0g

STRAWBERRY PIE

VEGETARIAN | GRAIN-FREE | GLUTEN-FREE | NUT-FREE | SOY-FREE | KID-FRIENDLY

Making a gluten-free pie crust that tastes good is, thankfully, not that difficult. This coconut flour, butter, and egg crust is firm and flavorful, and forms the perfect foundation for the fresh strawberry filling. Sugar is used in this recipe to sweeten the strawberries, making it most appropriate for Phase 2.

MAKES 1 PIE

Prep time: 15 minutes
Cook time: 15 minutes, plus
   2 hours chilling

For the crust

½ cup butter, melted; reserve the
   butter wrapper to grease the
   pie pan
2 large eggs
2 tablespoons granulated cane sugar
¼ teaspoon sea salt
¾ cup coconut flour

For the filling

4 cups strawberries, hulled and
   sliced, divided
1 cup water, divided
1 teaspoon fresh lemon juice
1 cup granulated cane sugar
2 tablespoons arrowroot powder

To make the crust

1. Preheat the oven to 400°F.

2. Grease a 9-inch pie pan with the reserved butter wrapper.

3. In a medium bowl, beat together the butter, eggs, sugar, and sea salt.

4. Add the coconut flour and mix until a sticky dough forms (it should hold together when pressed).

5. Press the dough into the bottom and sides of the prepared. Using a fork, poke about 20 sets of holes in the crust's surface.

6. Bake in the preheated oven for 10 minutes until golden brown. Remove from the oven and let cool.

To make the filling

1. Preheat the oven to 350°F.

2. In a saucepan over medium heat, combine 1 cup of strawberries and ½ cup of water, and simmer for 2 to 3 minutes until the berries begin to soften.

3. In another medium bowl, combine the remaining 3 cups of strawberries and the lemon juice, and toss to combine.

4. Pour half of the lemon-juice coated strawberries into the pie shell (you should be left with about 1½ cups of berries in the bowl).

5. To the remaining strawberries in the bowl, add the remaining ½ cup of water, the sugar, and arrowroot powder. Gently stir to mix well. Add this mixture to the saucepan and cook for 2 to 3 minutes, stirring constantly until it begins to thicken.

6. Pour the thickened strawberries over the strawberries in the pie shell. Bake in the preheated oven for 5 minutes. Remove from the oven and cool. Refrigerate for at least 2 hours to set. Serve cold.

PER SERVING: (1/6 pie) Calories: 365, Protein: 3g, Cholesterol: 95mg, Sodium: 212mg, Total Carbohydrates: 47g, Fiber: 3g, Total Fat: 21g, Saturated Fat: 13g

Ingredient Tip: To grease the pie pan, use the butter wrapper from the stick of butter to get the job done. It will have enough residual butter left on it to grease the pie dish.

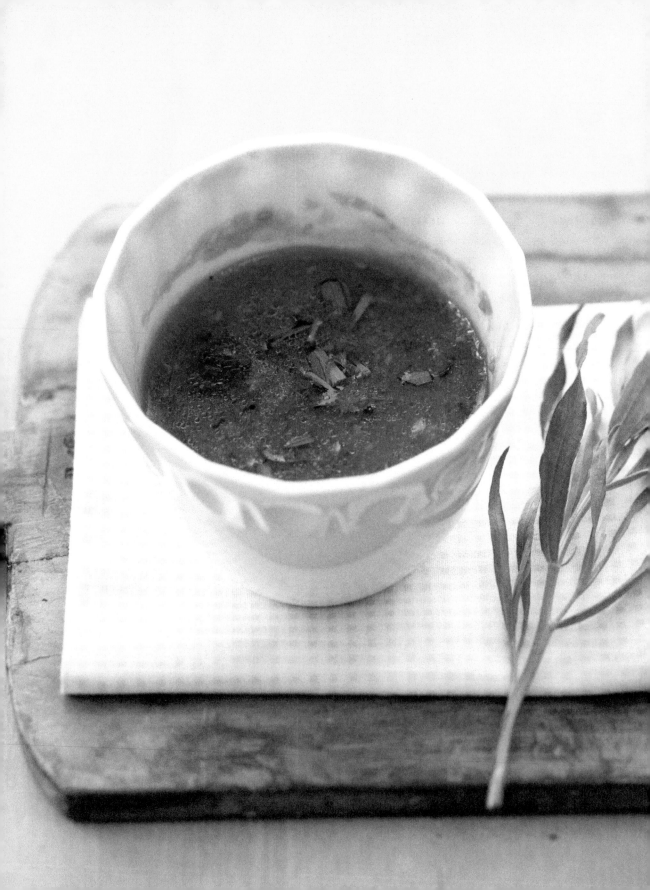

CONDIMENTS, DRESSINGS & SAUCES

The bad news is that you are unlikely to find both allium- and sugar-free condiments, dressings, and sauces at your local grocery store. The good news is that these items are all fairly easy to make at home. With just a few ingredients and a little bit of time, you can whip up many healthier and delicious accompaniments for serving with all of your favorite dishes.

RANCH-STYLE DRESSING

VEGETARIAN | GRAIN-FREE | GLUTEN-FREE | NUT-FREE | SOY-FREE |
KID-FRIENDLY | LOW-FODMAP

If you love ranch dressing, giving it up can be a tough adjustment. Purchased ranch is filled with garlic and onion, as well as many preservatives and fillers you should avoid. Try this fresh, yogurt-based version and you'll never go back.

MAKES 1½ CUPS

Prep time: 5 minutes

---

1 cup plain yogurt (not fat-free;
    see page 258)

½ cup mayonnaise

1 tablespoon dried parsley

1 teaspoon dried chives

1 teaspoon dried dill

½ teaspoon sea salt

¼ teaspoon freshly ground
    black pepper

*Phase 2 Tip: If tolerated, add
2 cloves of finely minced garlic
for even more flavor.*

In a small bowl, whisk together the yogurt, mayonnaise, parsley, chives, dill, sea salt, and pepper. Refrigerate in an airtight container for up to 5 days.

PER SERVING: (2T) Calories: 27, Protein: <1G, Cholesterol: 2mg, Sodium: 81mg, Total Carbohydrates: 2g, Fiber: 0g, Total Fat: 2g, Saturated Fat: 0g

MAPLE-MUSTARD DRESSING

VEGAN | GRAIN-FREE | GLUTEN-FREE | NUT-FREE | SOY-FREE | KID-FRIENDLY | LOW-FODMAP

Dijon mustard and maple syrup combine in this sweet and tangy dressing that pairs well with flavorful cheeses such as feta, Gorgonzola, and blue.

MAKES ABOUT ¾ CUP

Prep time: 5 minutes

¼ cup fresh lemon juice
¼ cup extra virgin olive oil
2 tablespoons pure maple syrup
1 tablespoon Dijon mustard
Sea salt
Freshly ground black pepper

Phase 2 Tip: If tolerated, add 2 cloves of finely minced garlic for even more flavor.

In a small bowl, whisk together the lemon juice, olive oil, maple syrup, and Dijon mustard. Season to taste with sea salt and pepper. Refrigerate in an airtight container for up to 5 days.

PER SERVING: (2T) Calories: 47, Protein: <1g, Cholesterol: 0mg, Sodium: 55mg, Total Carbohydrates: 2g, Fiber: 0g, Total Fat: 4g, Saturated Fat: <1g

RASPBERRY VINAIGRETTE

VEGAN | GRAIN-FREE | GLUTEN-FREE | NUT-FREE | SOY-FREE | KID-FRIENDLY | LOW-FODMAP

When raspberries are in season, the world gets a little sweeter. Make this dressing using fresh or frozen raspberries and enjoy the sweet treat on your salads all year long.

MAKES 1½ CUPS

Prep time: 10 minutes
Cook time: 5 minutes

---

1 cup fresh or frozen raspberries, thawed if frozen
¼ cup water
½ cup extra virgin olive oil
¼ cup red wine vinegar
¼ cup pure maple syrup
1 teaspoon Dijon mustard
¼ teaspoon sea salt
¼ teaspoon freshly ground black pepper

Phase 2 Tip: If tolerated, add 2 cloves of finely minced garlic for even more flavor.

1. In a small saucepan over medium heat, combine the raspberries and water and bring to a boil. Reduce the heat to low and simmer for 5 minutes. Using a fine-mesh strainer, strain the pulp from the liquid, pressing down with the back of a spoon to press as much liquid through as possible; set aside to cool. Discard the solids.

2. In a small bowl, whisk together the olive oil, red wine vinegar, maple syrup, Dijon mustard, sea salt, and pepper.

3. Add the strained raspberry juice and whisk well. Refrigerate in an airtight container for up to 5 days.

PER SERVING: (2T) Calories: 48, Protein: <1g, Cholesterol: 0mg, Sodium: 22mg, Total Carbohydrates: 3g, Fiber: 0mg, Total Fat: 4g, Saturated Fat: <1g

TARTAR SAUCE

VEGETARIAN | GRAIN-FREE | NUT-FREE | SOY-FREE | KID-FRIENDLY | LOW-FODMAP

Tartar sauce and fish are a beloved combination. Try this sauce with our Crunchy Oven-Baked Whitefish (page 162), or spread it on a sandwich. Either way, this simple condiment is best when made using homemade relish, which is free of high-fructose corn syrup, onions, and garlic.

MAKES ABOUT ¾ CUP

Prep time: 5 minutes

½ cup **mayonnaise**

3 tablespoons **Sweet Pickled Relish (page 247)**

Ingredient Tip: Many types of mayonnaise contain soybean oil, something that should be avoided during Phase 1; be sure to read the label. Also, some vinegars in mayonnaise are derived from wheat-based grains, so if you are sensitive to gluten, be wary. Many big-name brands both use corn-based vinegars in their mayonnaise.

In a small bowl, whisk together the mayonnaise and relish. Refrigerate in an airtight container for up to 5 days.

PER SERVING: (2T) Calories: 43, Protein: <1g, Cholesterol: 3mg, Sodium: 100mg, Total Carbohydrates: 4g, Fiber: 0g, Total Fat: 3g, Saturated Fat: 0g

ASIAN-STYLE CHILE SAUCE

VEGAN | GLUTEN-FREE | NUT-FREE | SOY-FREE | LOW-FODMAP

Most Asian-style chile sauces contain garlic, making them unsuitable for Phase 1 of this diet—but not this version. Use any red chile that suits your tastes. Red Thai chiles and habaneros are some of the hottest varieties. If desired, you can combine them with milder chiles, such as Fresnos, to tone down the heat.

MAKES ½ CUP

Prep time: 5 minutes
Cook time: 5 minutes

6 ounces hot chile peppers
(cayenne, Thai, habanero,
jalapeño, serrano)
2 tablespoons white vinegar
1 tablespoon pure maple syrup
½ teaspoon sea salt

Phase 2 Tip: Substitute 1 tablespoon of granulated sugar for the maple syrup, if desired.

Ingredient Tip: Ensure that the white vinegar you purchase is gluten-free and not made from grain. Many brands are distilled from corn.

1. In a food processor fitted with the metal blade, combine the chiles, white vinegar, maple syrup, and sea salt. Process just until chunky. Transfer to a small saucepan over medium heat.

2. Bring to a simmer and cook for 5 minutes, stirring frequently. Taste and adjust the seasonings, if desired. Cool completely, then refrigerate in an airtight container for up to 5 days.

PER SERVING: (2T) Calories: 14, Protein: <1g, Cholesterol: 0mg, Sodium: 118mg, Total Carbohydrates: 3g, Fiber: <1g, Total Fat: <1g, Saturated Fat: 0g

ALLIUM-FREE MARINARA SAUCE

VEGAN | GRAIN-FREE | GLUTEN-FREE | NUT-FREE | SOY-FREE | KID-FRIENDLY | LOW-FODMAP

Onion and garlic seem to be a staple in this classic sauce. Here, we reboot it without either ingredient, with great results. Enjoy it on pastas, meats, and vegetables.

MAKES ABOUT 1½ QUARTS

Prep time: 10 minutes
Cook time: 45 minutes

3 teaspoons extra virgin olive
   oil, divided
1 red bell pepper, finely diced
3 (15-ounce) cans diced tomatoes
¼ cup tightly packed fresh
   basil leaves
1 teaspoon pure maple syrup
1 teaspoon dried oregano
½ teaspoon sea salt
1 bay leaf
Freshly ground black pepper

Ingredient Tip: This sauce freezes well, so double the recipe and freeze the leftovers in an airtight container for a quick meal down the line.

1. In a medium saucepan over medium heat, heat 1 teaspoon of olive oil. Add the red bell pepper and sauté for about 5 minutes until slightly browned and beginning to soften.

2. Stir in the tomatoes, basil, maple syrup, oregano, sea salt, and bay leaf. Season to taste with pepper and bring to a boil. Reduce the heat to low and simmer for 30 to 40 minutes, stirring about every 10 minutes until slightly thickened. Remove from the heat and let cool.

3. Remove the bay leaf and transfer the mixture to a blender and purée until smooth. Taste and adjust the seasonings, if desired.

PER SERVING: (per cup) Calories: 51, Protein: 2g, Cholesterol: 0mg, Sodium: 126mg, Total Carbohydrates: 8g Fiber: 2g, Total Fat: 2g, Saturated Fat: 0g

SUGAR-FREE KETCHUP

VEGAN | DAIRY-FREE | GRAIN-FREE | GLUTEN-FREE | NUT-FREE | SOY-FREE |
KID-FRIENDLY | LOW-FODMAP

Purchased ketchup typically contains high-fructose corn syrup, garlic, and onions. Thankfully, it's easy to avoid those ingredients without sacrificing the flavor of the real thing. Here, tomato paste and traditional spices yield a thick and well-balanced ketchup.

MAKES ABOUT 2 CUPS

Prep time: 10 minutes

---

1 (12-ounce) can tomato paste
½ cup water
¼ cup apple cider vinegar
3 tablespoons pure maple syrup
½ teaspoon ground mustard seeds
½ teaspoon sea salt
½ teaspoon ground cinnamon
½ teaspoon ground cloves
¼ teaspoon ground
    asafetida powder

Phase 2 Tip: For a richer flavor, substitute an equal amount of dark brown sugar for the maple syrup.

In a small bowl, whisk together the tomato paste, water, apple cider vinegar, maple syrup, mustard seeds, sea salt, cinnamon, cloves, and asafetida. Refrigerate in an airtight container for up to 3 weeks.

PER SERVING: (2T) Calories: 14, Protein: <1g, Cholesterol: 0mg, Sodium: 42mg, Total Carbohydrates: 3g, Fiber: 0mg, Total Fat: <1g, Saturated Fat: 0g

RASPBERRY-CHIA JAM

VEGAN | DAIRY-FREE | GRAIN-FREE | GLUTEN-FREE | NUT-FREE | SOY-FREE | KID-FRIENDLY | LOW-FODMAP

If you are familiar with chia seeds, you'll know they become gel-like when mixed with liquid. This makes chia a perfect substitute for pectin in jam making. Jams made with chia also don't require extra sugar to help them set, so you can sweeten simply with a bit of maple syrup. Use fresh or frozen berries for this quick jam, and spoon it over pancakes, waffles, or a piece of toast for a delicious sweet treat.

MAKES ½ CUP

Prep time: 5 minutes
Cook time: 20 minutes

1 cup fresh or frozen raspberries
1½ tablespoons pure maple syrup
1 tablespoon chia seeds

Ingredient Tip: Fresh raspberries are very easy to freeze. Simply rinse the berries and arrange them in a single layer on a baking sheet. Freeze until solid, and then transfer them to an airtight container; they'll keep, frozen, for up to 1 year.

1. In a small saucepan, combine the berries and the maple syrup. Bring to a boil, reduce the heat to low, and simmer for 10 minutes, stirring constantly.

2. Using a potato masher or large fork, smash the berries in the pan. Cook for 5 minutes more.

3. Add the chia seeds and cook for 3 to 5 minutes, stirring constantly until the jam is thickened. Let cool, then transfer to a small airtight container. Cover and refrigerate for up to 10 days.

PER SERVING: (2T) Calories: 52, Protein: 2g, Cholesterol: 0mg, Sodium: 2mg, Total Carbohydrates: 13g, Fiber:2g , Total Fat: 1g, Saturated Fat: 0g

STRAWBERRY SHORTCAKE SYRUP

VEGETARIAN | GRAIN-FREE | GLUTEN-FREE | NUT-FREE | SOY-FREE |
KID-FRIENDLY | LOW-FODMAP

Turn up your breakfast game with this sweet fruit syrup, which is higher in fiber than plain maple syrup thanks to the strawberries. Pour it over pancakes, waffles, and crêpes or layer it in parfaits along with plain yogurt, fruit, and granola.

SERVES 4

Prep time: 10 minutes
Cook time: 5 minutes

2 cups fresh or frozen strawberries
¼ cup water
½ teaspoon orange zest
1 tablespoon fresh orange juice
1 tablespoon pure maple syrup
1 teaspoon pure vanilla extract
3 tablespoons plain yogurt (not fat-free)

Cooking Tip: An immersion blender works best to purée this sauce; simply submerge the blender into the slightly cooled sauce and blend.

1. In a saucepan over medium heat, combine the strawberries, water, orange zest, orange juice, and maple syrup and bring to a boil. Boil for about 5 minutes until the mixture has thickened slightly. Remove from the heat and let cool slightly.

2. Using an immersion blender or regular blender, purée until smooth. Add the vanilla and yogurt and pulse just to combine.

3. Transfer to an airtight container and refrigerate for up to 3 days.

PER SERVING: Calories: 49, Protein: 2g, Cholesterol: 1mg, Sodium: 157mg, Total Carbohydrates: 10g, Fiber: 1g, Total Fat: <1g, Saturated Fat: 0g

SESAME-SOY DIPPING SAUCE

VEGAN | DAIRY-FREE | GRAIN-FREE | NUT-FREE | KID-FRIENDLY | LOW-FODMAP

This Asian-inspired dipping sauce pairs well with both shrimp and fish. Serve it with Coconut Shrimp (page 164) or Crunchy Oven-Baked Whitefish (page 162) as an alternative to Tartar Sauce (page 226). Adjust the level of heat by using more or less chile, as desired.

MAKES ABOUT ¼ CUP

Prep time: 10 minutes

¼ cup soy sauce

2 teaspoons pure maple syrup

1 tablespoon sesame oil

2 teaspoons rice vinegar

2 scallions (green part
　　only), minced

1 serrano chile pepper, seeded
　　and minced

Ingredient Tip: Soy sauce is low in FODMAPs, so you can enjoy it in both Phase 1 and Phase 2 of the Microbiome Diet. However, if you avoid gluten, substitute gluten-free tamari in any of the recipes that call for soy sauce.

In a small bowl, whisk together the soy sauce, maple syrup, sesame oil, rice vinegar, scallion greens, and chile. Cover and refrigerate until ready to use.

PER SERVING: Calories: 52, Protein: 2g, Cholesterol: 0mg, Sodium: 900mg, Total Carbohydrates: 4g, Fiber: <1g, Total Fat: 3g, Saturated Fat: 0g

THAI-STYLE PEANUT DIPPING SAUCE

VEGAN | DAIRY-FREE | GRAIN-FREE | KID-FRIENDLY | LOW-FODMAP

This protein-packed sauce is really versatile: Use it as a dip for fresh veggies (carrots, celery, broccoli, cauliflower), or over grilled meat (pork, chicken, and even beef), or toss it with shredded kale or cabbage for an easy Asian-inspired salad.

MAKES ABOUT 1¾ CUPS

Prep time: 10 minutes

----

1 cup smooth peanut butter

¼ cup soy sauce

¼ cup rice vinegar

¼ cup water

2 tablespoons lime juice

1 tablespoon sesame oil

3 scallions (green part only), minced

Ingredient Tip: If all you have on hand is chunky peanut butter, that's fine, too. Combine the ingredients in a blender or food processor and process until smooth.

In a small bowl, whisk together the peanut butter, soy sauce, rice vinegar, water, lime juice, and sesame oil. Serve, garnished with the scallion greens. The sauce will keep refrigerated in an airtight container for up to 3 days.

PER SERVING: (2T) Calories: 62, Protein: 3g, Cholesterol: 0mg, Sodium: 171mg, Total Carbohydrates: 2g, Fiber: <1g, Total Fat: 5g, Saturated Fat: 1g

CHIMICHURRI SAUCE

VEGAN | DAIRY-FREE | GRAIN-FREE | GLUTEN-FREE | NUT-FREE | SOY-FREE |
KID-FRIENDLY | LOW-FODMAP

Chimichurri sauce originates from Argentina, where it is slathered on roasted meats like butter on bread. It is a simple and bright sauce packed with herbs. It leaves a wonderful, palate-cleansing flavor in the mouth. Toss the sauce with vegetables, noodles, or meat for a quick and savory addition to your table.

MAKES ABOUT ½ CUP

Prep time: 10 minutes

½ cup chopped fresh flat-leaf Italian parsley leaves

¼ cup chopped fresh cilantro leaves

5 scallions (green part only), minced

2 tablespoons red wine vinegar

¼ teaspoon red pepper flakes

½ cup extra virgin olive oil

Sea salt

Freshly ground black pepper

Variation Tip: Play around with different ratios of parsley and cilantro based on your preferences. In Phase 2, you can add 2 or 3 cloves of crushed garlic.

In a food processor fitted with the metal blade, pulse to combine the parsley, cilantro, scallion greens, red wine vinegar, and red pepper flakes. While the motor is running, gradually add the olive oil and process until smooth. Season to taste with sea salt and pepper. The sauce will keep refrigerated in an airtight container for up to 3 days.

PER SERVING: (2T) Calories: 113, Protein: <1g, Cholesterol: 0mg, Sodium: 63mg, Total Carbohydrates: 1g, Fiber: 0g, Total Fat: 13g, Saturated Fat: 2g

SUN-DRIED TOMATO-BASIL CREAM CHEESE

VEGETARIAN | GRAIN-FREE | GLUTEN-FREE | NUT-FREE | SOY-FREE | KID-FRIENDLY | LOW-FODMAP

Savory sun-dried tomatoes and fragrant basil elevate this simple cream cheese spread. Spread on some gluten-free crackers or bread for a flavorful and satiating midday snack. In Phase 2, smear it on some celery for a light snack.

MAKES 1 CUP

Prep time: 10 minutes

---

1 (8-ounce) package cream cheese, at room temperature

½ cup chopped sun-dried tomatoes (packed in oil)

2 tablespoons finely sliced fresh basil

Variation Tip: For the same flavor but about two-thirds less fat, try substituting an equal quantity of Neufchâtel cheese for the cream cheese.

In a small bowl, stir together the cream cheese, sun-dried tomatoes, and basil using a rubber spatula. Transfer to an airtight container and refrigerate for up to 5 days.

PER SERVING: (2T) Calories: 51, Protein: 1g, Cholesterol: 16mg, Sodium: 42mg, Total Carbohydrates: <1g, Fiber: 0g, Total Fat: 5g, Saturated Fat: 3g

OLIVE TAPENADE

VEGAN | DAIRY-FREE | GRAIN-FREE | GLUTEN-FREE | NUT-FREE | SOY-FREE |
KID-FRIENDLY | LOW-FODMAP

Olive tapenade is an easy way to lend Mediterranean flair to so many foods. Use it as a savory dip for veggies and crackers or pita, as a zesty alternative to mayonnaise on sandwiches, or even as a topping for fish and chicken.

MAKES 1 CUP

Prep time: 5 minutes

---

1 cup pitted Kalamata olives
2 tablespoons chopped fresh
    flat-leaf Italian parsley leaves
2 fresh basil leaves
2 tablespoons fresh lemon juice
2 tablespoons extra virgin olive oil
1 tablespoon capers, drained

Phase 2 Tip: If tolerated, add 1 to 2 crushed garlic cloves for even more flavor.

In a food processor fitted with the metal blade, combine the olives, parsley, basil, lemon juice, olive oil, and capers and process to a coarse paste. Transfer to an airtight container and refrigerate for up to 5 days.

PER SERVING: (2T) Calories: 25, Protein: <1g, Cholesterol: 0mg, Sodium: 90mg, Total Carbohydrates: <1g, Fiber: 0g, Total Fat: 3g, Saturated Fat: 0g

YOGURT TAHINI SAUCE

VEGETARIAN | GRAIN-FREE | GLUTEN-FREE | NUT-FREE | SOY-FREE | KID-FRIENDLY

This recipe combines yogurt with purchased tahini for an easy probiotic boost loaded with healthy fats thanks to the sesame seeds in the tahini. You can find jars or cans of tahini in most grocery stores in the same section as peanut butter, or with Middle Eastern foods. Scoop a spoonful of this tahini sauce on salads or serve it as a dipping sauce with the Parmesan-Quinoa Patties (page 116).

MAKES 1 HEAPING CUP

Prep time: 5 minutes

¾ **cup plain yogurt (not fat-free)**
¼ **cup tahini**
1½ **tablespoons fresh lemon juice**
½ **teaspoon sea salt**

Phase 2 Tip: If tolerated, add 1 to 2 minced garlic cloves for even more flavor.

In a small bowl, whisk together the yogurt, tahini, lemon juice, and sea salt. Transfer to an airtight container and refrigerate for up to 5 days.

PER SERVING: (2T) Calories: 31, Protein: 1g, Cholesterol: 1mg, Sodium: 71mg, Total Carbohydrates: 2g, Fiber: 0g, Total Fat: 2g, Saturated Fat: 0g

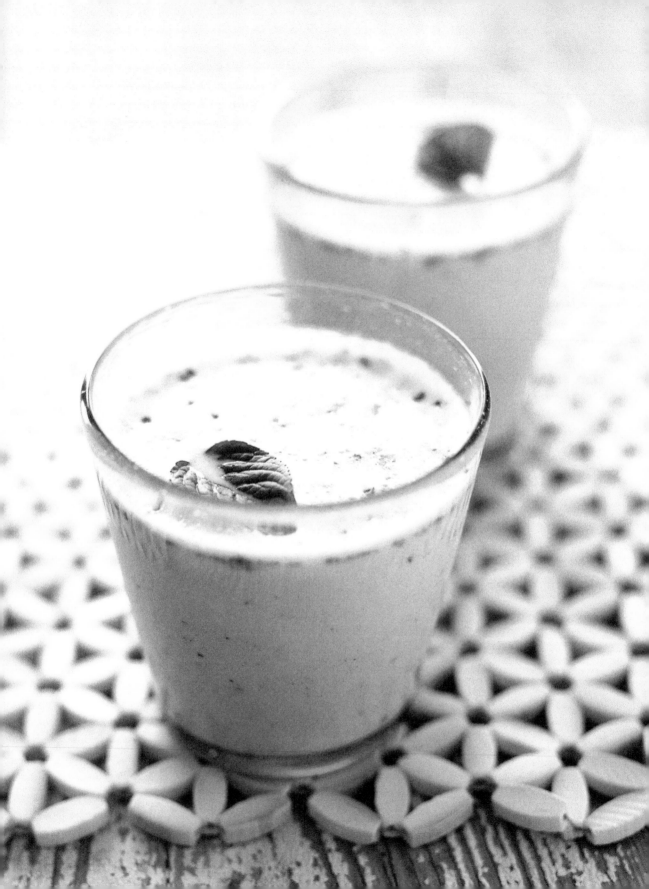

FERMENTED FOODS & DRINKS

Consuming fermented foods and drinks as part of your daily routine is a cornerstone of the Microbiome Diet. While purchased fermented foods save time, it's easy to make them yourself at home, which also saves money. Practiced for centuries throughout the world, fermenting is a fun way to use up and store produce, and the results can help heal your body and set you on a path of weight loss and improved health and digestion.

IS THIS SAFE?

Fermentation is a safe process when you take the necessary precautions and follow the salt-to-water ratios outlined in these recipes. If this is your first time fermenting, before beginning any fermentation project, review the introduction to fermentation on pages 56–57. While there are things that can go wrong, it is pretty easy to produce a ferment on your own—even your first time. As with other foods, your nose is the best judge as to whether a fermented food has gone bad. You don't want to eat anything that looks or smells bad, but chances are, this will not happen on your first, fifth, or even twentieth ferment. Signs of spoilage in vegetable ferments include sliminess, rancid smells, and rot. If these instances occur, discard the foods without tasting them.

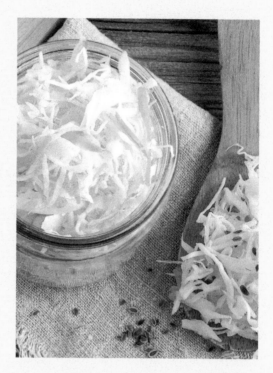

In lactic acid fermentation, salt is not a starter culture, but rather a protectant. When foods are properly salted, the salt protects the food from spoilage bacteria, while the good bacteria are able to gain hold and reproduce. As the bacteria eat and digest the naturally occurring sugars in produce, they create lactic acid, which is responsible for the sour taste of fermented foods. Once fully fermented, there is enough lactic acid present to prevent spoilage in the finished product. After fermentation is complete, all fermented foods should be refrigerated to halt fermentation.

SAUERKRAUT

VEGAN | DAIRY-FREE | GRAIN-FREE | GLUTEN-FREE | NUT-FREE | SOY-FREE |
KID-FRIENDLY | LOW-FODMAP

This is a great project for a first-time fermenter. The ingredients are inexpensive, no special equipment is required, and the task is rather simple. The recipe makes a small batch, just enough to fit in a quart jar. Once accustomed to the process, you can easily double or triple this recipe to make a larger batch.

MAKES 1 QUART

Prep time: 10 minutes
Fermentation time: 2 to 6 weeks

½ **small head cabbage**
    (about 1¼ pounds)
1½ **teaspoons pickling salt**

1. Using a sharp knife, remove the cabbage core. Remove and reserve 2 of the outer cabbage leaves. Using a sharp knife or mandolin, thinly shred the cabbage into ¼-inch strips.

2. In a medium nonreactive bowl, combine the cabbage and pickling salt. Using your hands, massage the salt into the cabbage. Let sit for 10 minutes, or until the cabbage begins to release its juices.

3. Pack the cabbage tightly into a wide-mouthed quart jar, pressing down firmly with a clean hand as you go. Place the reserved leaves on top of the cabbage to hold it down.

4. Fill a narrow glass jelly jar with water and affix its lid. Place the filled jar into the opening of the wide-mouth jar to act as a weight. Press down on it firmly. Cover the jars with a clean kitchen towel secured with a rubber band and set aside in a cool location away from direct sunlight.

5. After 24 hours, the amount of brine produced by the cabbage should cover the cabbage. If it doesn't, mix 2 cups of water with 2 teaspoons of pickling salt and stir to dissolve. Pour this brine over the cabbage so it is completely submerged and weigh it down with the smaller water-filled jar.

6. Check the cabbage daily for scum forming on the surface. If any scum appears on the sauerkraut, skim it off using a clean nonreactive spoon. Remove and rinse the outside of the water-filled jar, as well. Replace the water-filled jar to reweight the cabbage, and cover it with a clean kitchen towel.

7. After 2 weeks, taste the sauerkraut. Once you are satisfied with the flavor, which can take up to 6 weeks, end active fermentation by removing the weight, placing a lid on the quart jar, and transferring it to the refrigerator.

PER SERVING: (1 cup) Calories: 18, Protein: 1g, Cholesterol: 0mg, Sodium: 733mg, Total Carbohydrates: 4g, Fiber: 2g, Total Fat: <1g, Saturated Fat: 0mg,

Variation Tip: For a bit of color, use a mix of white and red cabbage. If desired, add ½ teaspoon of dried spices such as dill, fennel, coriander, or caraway seeds. A sliced hot chile or a few slices of peeled ginger can also add a nice flavor.

CURTIDO

VEGAN | DAIRY-FREE | GRAIN-FREE | GLUTEN-FREE | NUT-FREE | SOY-FREE | KID-FRIENDLY | LOW-FODMAP

Curtido is a spicy, Latin American take on sauerkraut. Similar to coleslaw, this fiery mix is fermented for only a couple of days so the cabbage retains much of its characteristic crunch.

MAKES 1 QUART

Prep time: 10 minutes, plus
  1 hour resting
Fermentation time: 3 days

1 small head cabbage (about
    1½ pounds)
8 scallions (green part only)
2 carrots, grated
2 tablespoons chopped
    fresh cilantro
1 serrano chile, minced
½ teaspoon red pepper flakes
¾ teaspoon pickling salt
¼ cup white wine vinegar

Phase 2 Tip: Add ½ red onion, thinly sliced, to the mixture in step 2.

1. Using a sharp knife, core the cabbage and cut it into quarters. Using a sharp knife or mandolin, cut each quarter into ¼-inch strips.

2. In a large bowl, combine the cabbage, scallion greens, carrots, cilantro, chile, red pepper flakes, and pickling salt. Stir to mix well. Cover the bowl with a clean kitchen towel and set aside for 1 hour at room temperature.

3. Fill a narrow glass jelly jar with water and affix its lid.

4. Pack the cabbage mixture tightly into a quart jar, pressing down firmly with a clean hand as you go. Add any liquid from the bowl to the jar, as well as the white wine vinegar.

5. Press the vegetables down below the brine, and place the water-filled jar in the mouth of the quart jar to act as a weight. Cover the jars with a clean kitchen towel secured with a rubber band and leave it at room temperature for 2 days.

6. Remove the weight and seal the jar with the lid. Refrigerate for up to 3 weeks.

PER SERVING: (1 cup) Calories: 54, Protein: 2g, Cholesterol: 0mg, Sodium: 409mg, Total Carbohydrates: 12g, Fiber: 4g, Total Fat: <1g, Saturated Fat: 0g

KIMCHI

VEGAN | DAIRY-FREE | GRAIN-FREE | GLUTEN-FREE | NUT-FREE | SOY-FREE | KID-FRIENDLY | LOW-FODMAP

Kimchi, a Korean version of sauerkraut, has a distinct and noteworthy taste due to the inclusion of ginger and hot peppers. Left to ferment for only a few days to a week, kimchi is much less sour than other fermented cabbage dishes, and also uses the more tender napa cabbage.

MAKES 1 QUART

Prep time: 10 minutes, plus
  12 hours resting
Fermentation time: 3 to 6 days

---

1 small head napa cabbage (about
  1½ pounds)
2 tablespoons plus ¾ teaspoon
  pickling salt, divided
4 cups water
8 scallions (green part only),
  sliced thinly
1 tablespoon peeled fresh
  ginger, minced
1 teaspoon ground paprika
¾ teaspoon sugar
½ teaspoon cayenne pepper

Ingredient Tip: Cayenne pepper is not the traditional spicy agent used in kimchi. However, it is readily available, and, when used with paprika, mimics the hue and flavor of the Korean ground peppers traditionally used. If you have access to Korean ground peppers, which are significantly milder than cayenne, substitute 1½ teaspoons for the cayenne and paprika.

1. Using a sharp knife, remove the cabbage core. Cut the leaves into 2-inch pieces.

2. In a large bowl (big enough to hold the cabbage), dissolve 2 tablespoons of pickling salt in the water.

3. Add the cabbage and use a large plate to weigh it below the brine. Cover the bowl with a clean kitchen towel, and set aside at room temperature for 12 hours.

4. The next day, strain the cabbage and reserve the brine. Return the cabbage to the bowl. Add the remaining ¾ teaspoon of pickling salt and the remaining ingredients. Stir well to combine.

5. Pack the cabbage tightly into a quart jar, pressing down firmly with a clean hand as you go. Cover the cabbage completely with the reserved brine.

6. Pour the remaining brine into a clean food-safe resealable bag, and stuff this bag into the opening of the jar. Place the jar on a plate to catch any dripping brine, and leave to ferment in a cool location for 3 to 6 days. Taste the kimchi after 3 days. When it is to your liking, remove the brine bag, affix a lid, and refrigerate it for several months.

PER SERVING: (1 cup) Calories: 33, Protein: 2g,
Cholesterol: 0mg, Sodium: 3,321mg, Total Carbohydrates: 7g,
Fiber: 2g, Total Fat: <1g, Saturated Fat: 0g

RADISH KIMCHI

VEGAN | DAIRY-FREE | GRAIN-FREE | GLUTEN-FREE | NUT-FREE | SOY-FREE |
KID-FRIENDLY | LOW-FODMAP

Radish adds such a lovely crunch to kimchi, and because radish is a known digestive aid, this is a perfect kimchi to have alongside a heavy, fatty meal. Eat radishes and radish kimchi at the end of a meal to aid digestion. A mix of French and red radishes provides a balanced, mellower flavor. If French radishes are unavailable, use 2 bunches of red radishes instead.

MAKES 1 QUART

Prep time: 10 minutes,
   plus 12 hours resting
Fermentation time: 3 to 6 days

---

2 tablespoons pickling salt, divided

4 cups water

1 bunch red radishes, ends trimmed
   and cut into ½-inch cubes

1 bunch French radishes, ends
   trimmed and cut into
   ½-inch cubes

8 scallions (green part only), sliced

1 tablespoon peeled fresh
   ginger, minced

1½ teaspoons paprika

¾ teaspoon cayenne pepper

¾ teaspoon granulated sugar

Variation Tip: The root and top ends of the radishes are edible and taste good, so, if you like, just give them a good washing and ferment them, too. To do this, cut the radishes lengthwise through the greens so each piece has a bit of green top still attached.

1. In a large bowl, (big enough to hold all the radishes), dissolve 1 tablespoon and 2 teaspoons of pickling salt in the water. Add the radishes, and place a large plate on top to hold the radishes below the brine. Cover the bowl with a clean kitchen towel, and set aside at room temperature for 12 hours.

2. The following day, using a colander, strain the radishes and reserve the brine. Return the radishes to the bowl, and add the remaining 1 teaspoon of pickling salt, the scallion greens, ginger, paprika, cayenne pepper, and sugar. Stir well.

3. Pack the radishes tightly into a quart jar, pressing down firmly with a clean hand as you go. Pour enough of the reserved brine over the radishes to cover completely.

4. Pour the remaining brine into a clean food-safe resealable plastic bag, and stuff this bag into the opening of the jar. Place the jar on a plate to catch any dripping brine, and leave to ferment in a cool location for 3 to 6 days. Taste the kimchi after 3 days. When it is to your liking, remove the brine bag, affix a lid, and refrigerate for several months.

PER SERVING: (per cup) Calories: 39, Protein: 2g, Cholesterol: 0mg, Sodium: 2,938mg, Total Carbohydrates: 9g, Fiber: 3g, Total Fat: <1g, Saturated Fat: 0g

SWEET PICKLED RELISH

VEGETARIAN | GRAIN-FREE | GLUTEN-FREE | NUT-FREE | SOY-FREE |
KID FRIENDLY | LOW-FODMAP

Great on hot sandwiches and a necessary component of tartar sauce, sweet pickled relish is a simple and fun ferment. This recipe uses whey, a by-product of cheese making, to get the fermentation process started. To obtain whey from kefir or yogurt, line a wire mesh strainer with a couple layers of coffee filters and pour the kefir or yogurt into the strainer, letting the liquid whey drain out into a jar below. Refrigerated any unused whey in an airtight jar for up to 2 weeks.

MAKES 1 PINT

Prep time: 10 minutes
Fermentation time: 3 days

---

2 cups finely chopped cucumbers
¼ cup finely chopped red
    bell pepper
¼ cup finely chopped scallions
    (green part only)
1½ teaspoons celery seeds
1 teaspoon yellow mustard seeds
¼ cup pure maple syrup
¾ teaspoon sea salt
½ teaspoon whey
½ teaspoon ground turmeric

*Phase 2 Tip: Add ½ red onion,
finely diced, in step 1 and omit
the scallion greens.*

1. In a small bowl, mix the cucumbers, red bell pepper, scallion greens, celery seeds, and mustard seeds. Pack tightly into a pint jar, pressing down firmly.

2. In the same bowl, mix the maple syrup, sea salt, whey, and turmeric. Pour this over the cucumbers, and, using a nonreactive spoon or clean hand, press the vegetables down below the liquid. Apply a weight (see page 242) to keep the vegetables below the surface of the liquid. Cover the jar tightly with a lid, and leave at room temperature to ferment for 3 days.

3. Remove the weight, reseal the jar, and transfer to the refrigerator where the relish will keep for 6 months.

PER SERVING: (2T) Calories: 9, Protein: 1g, T Cholesterol: 0mg, Sodium: 44mg, otal Carbohydrates: 3g, Fiber: 0g, Total Fat: <1g, Saturated Fat: 0g

PICKLED DAIKON

VEGAN | DAIRY-FREE | GRAIN-FREE | GLUTEN-FREE | NUT-FREE | SOY-FREE | KID-FRIENDLY | LOW-FODMAP

Like red radishes, the daikon radish contains digestive enzymes and is a diuretic. Here it is fermented for a light sour taste. If desired, add some red chili flakes or whole dried chiles, minced ginger, or whole peppercorns. When serving, trying sprinkling these pickles with a little Chinese five-spice powder for something different.

MAKES 1 QUART

Prep time: 10 minutes
Fermentation time: 2 to 5 days

1 pound daikon
1½ tablespoons pickling salt
2 cups water

Ingredient Tip: Daikon do not need to be peeled before using. Simply scrub the skin well using a clean brush to remove any surface dirt.

1. Using a sharp knife, cut the daikon into ¼-inch rounds and pack into a quart jar.

2. In a medium bowl, combine the pickling salt and water and stir until dissolved. Pour over the daikon. Use a weight to hold the daikon below the brine (see page 242). Close the jar loosely with a lid and set aside at room temperature for 2 to 5 days. Open the lid every day or two to release any built up gases.

3. Taste the daikon after 2 days. When it reaches the desired level of sourness, remove the weight, affix the lid, and refrigerate for up to 1 month.

PER SERVING: (per cup) Calories: 18, Protein: 1g, Cholesterol: 0mg, Sodium: 363mg, Total Carbohydrates: 4g, Fiber: 2g, Total Fat: <1g, Saturated Fat: 0g

DILL PICKLES

VEGAN | DAIRY-FREE | GRAIN-FREE | GLUTEN-FREE | NUT-FREE | SOY-FREE |
KID-FRIENDLY | LOW-FODMAP

Perhaps one of the most famous fermentations, the dill pickle is attainable even for the beginning fermenter. You will need to source some pickling cucumbers, a smaller, thicker-skinned variety than slicing cucumbers. Look for them, along with fresh dill heads in grocery stores and farm markets starting in midsummer.

MAKES 2 QUARTS

Prep time: 10 minutes
Fermentation time: 4 weeks

———

2½ pounds pickling cucumbers
3 to 5 fresh dill heads
1 dried chile, split lengthwise
½ teaspoon whole
　black peppercorns
3½ tablespoons pickling salt
5 cups water

1. Wash the cucumbers gently in cold water, and remove the blossom end. If desired, slice the cucumbers lengthwise in halves or quarters.

2. Pack the cucumbers, dill heads, chile, and peppercorns into a half-gallon jar, or divide between 2 quart-size jars.

3. In a large bowl, combine the water and pickling salt and stir until dissolved. Pour over the cucumbers. Use a small weight to hold the cucumbers below the brine (see page 242). Cover the jar with a clean kitchen towel secured with a rubber band, and set aside at room temperature.

4. After 2 or 3 days, you should see bubbles rising to the surface. Begin checking daily for scum forming on the surface. If any forms, use a nonreactive spoon to remove it promptly, then rinse the weight and return it to the jar.

5. Continue fermentation for about 4 weeks, or until the bubbles stop rising. Strain the pickles and reserve the brine. Remove and discard the dill heads, chile, and peppercorns. Rinse the pickles under cold water and drain. ▶

DILL PICKLES *continued*

Variation Tip: Removing the dill, chiles, and peppercorns and simmering the brine allows you to extend the shelf life of this product for up to 6 months. However, since you are making only a small amount of pickles, this may not be necessary: If you plan to use the pickles within 1 month, you can skip this step.

6. Transfer the brine to a small saucepan over medium-high heat and bring to a simmer. Cook for 5 minutes, skimming off any scum that rises to the top. Remove from the heat and let cool to room temperature.

7. Wash the jar with soap and water. Pack the pickles back into the clean jar. Pour the cooled brine over the pickles. Seal the jar with the lid and refrigerate for up to 6 months.

PER SERVING: (2 pickles) Calories: 40, Protein: 2g, Cholesterol: 0mg, Sodium: 363 mg Total Carbohydrates: 9g, Fiber: 2g, Total Fat: <1g, Saturated Fat: 0g

HOT & SPICY PICKLES

VEGAN | DAIRY-FREE | GRAIN-FREE | GLUTEN-FREE | NUT-FREE | SOY-FREE | KID-FRIENDLY | LOW-FODMAP

Mustard pickles are appealing in both appearance and flavor, and are super easy to make. Use yellow mustard seeds for the best color. Three chiles are recommended for the best heat level, but you can use more or less based on your preference.

MAKES 1 CUP

Prep time: 10 minutes
Fermentation time: 2 to 3 weeks

2½ pounds pickling cucumbers
2 tablespoons mustard seeds
3 fresh dill heads
3 dried red Thai chiles
3 tablespoons pickling salt
4 cups water

Ingredient Tip: Thai chiles are quite spicy and have a distinct flavor. If you don't have access to dried Thai chiles, use any other dried variety you choose (adjust the amount accordingly).

1. Wash the cucumbers gently in cold water, and remove the blossom end. If desired, slice the cucumbers lengthwise in halves or quarters.

2. Pack the cucumbers, mustard seeds, dill heads, and chiles into a half-gallon jar or 2 quart-size jars.

3. In a large bowl, combine the pickling salt and water and stir until dissolved. Pour the brine over the cucumbers. Use a small weight to hold the cucumbers below the brine (see page 242). Cover the jar with a clean kitchen towel and set aside at room temperature.

4. After 2 or 3 days, you should see bubbles rising to the surface. Begin checking daily for scum forming on the surface. If any forms, use a nonreactive spoon to remove it promptly, then rinse the weight and return it to the jar.

5. Continue fermentation for 2 or 3 weeks, or until the bubbles stop rising. Remove the weight, seal the jar with the lid, and refrigerate for up to 3 months.

PER SERVING: (1/4 cup) Calories: 80, Protein: 4g, Cholesterol: 0mg, Sodium: 636mg, Total Carbohydrates: 15g, Fiber: 3g, Total Fat: 2g, Saturated Fat: 0g

DILLY BEANS

VEGAN | DAIRY-FREE | GRAIN-FREE | GLUTEN-FREE | NUT-FREE | SOY-FREE | KID-FRIENDLY | LOW-FODMAP

Dilly beans are a quick side dish, great for snacking, and a lovely addition to a Bloody Mary drink. Here we use young green snap beans, but you can use whatever you have on hand. Dill is the star of the show here, but feel free to add your favorite herbs and spices.

MAKES 1 QUART

Prep time: 10 minutes
Fermentation time: 2 weeks

_____

½ **pound young snap beans, trimmed**
½ **teaspoon whole**
   black peppercorns
3 **fresh dill heads**
2 **tablespoons pickling salt**
3 **cups water**

Ingredient Tip: Like other fermentation recipes, other spices can be added. However, always use whole spices: Ground spices are more commonly contaminated with mold, which can lead to spoilage in your fermented foods.

1. Layer the beans, peppercorns, and dill heads in a quart jar.

2. In a small bowl, combine the pickling salt and water, stirring until the salt is dissolved. Pour the brine over the beans. Use a small weight to hold the beans below the surface (see page 242). Cover with a loose lid, airlock, or bag filled with brine (see page 245) and set aside at room temperature.

3. Within a few days, bubbles will begin rising to the surface. Check the jar daily for any scum on the surface. If any forms, use a nonreactive spoon to remove it promptly, then rinse the weight and return it to the jar.

4. In about 2 weeks fermentation will be complete, and bubbles will stop rising to the surface. Remove the weight, seal with the lid, and refrigerate for up to 1 month.

PER SERVING: Calories: ¼ cup, Protein: 6, Cholesterol: 0mg, Sodium: 363mg, Total Carbohydrates: 1g, Fiber: <1g, Total Fat: <1g, Saturated Fat: 0g

HONEY-FERMENTED GARLIC

VEGETARIAN | DAIRY-FREE | GRAIN-FREE | GLUTEN-FREE | NUT-FREE | SOY-FREE

Good-quality garlic is a must for this recipe; ensure the cloves are not dried or sprouting. The finished product can be used raw or cooked, and gives a deep, sweet-garlicky flavor to salad dressings, dips, and sauces. Try mixing the fermented garlic with soy sauce, ginger, and additional honey for an unforgettable chicken wing sauce.

MAKES ABOUT 1 PINT

Prep time: 15 minutes
Fermenting time: 4 weeks

---

5 small whole garlic bulbs, separated into cloves and peeled
2 cups unpasteurized raw honey

Cooking Tip: Experienced fermenters recommend leaving the garlic to ferment even longer that the 4 weeks—up to 1 year. At any point, some of the garlic can be removed with a clean spoon and consumed, leaving the remaining garlic to continue fermenting.

1. Place the garlic into a pint glass jar.

2. Pour in enough honey to cover the garlic completely, leaving about 2 inches of headspace at the top of the jar. Screw on the lid loosely.

3. Set the jar on a plate in a cool, dark place with a clean tea towel draped over top. Let it ferment for about 4 weeks, opening it daily to let out air. Ensure the garlic remains coated in honey by occasionally rolling the jar from side to side.

4. Once fermentation is complete, seal with the lid, and transfer to the refrigerator where it will last up to 1 year.

PER SERVING: (2T) Calories: 140, Protein: 1g, Cholesterol: 0mg, Sodium: 3mg, Total Carbohydrates: 37g, Fiber: 0g, Total Fat: 0g, Saturated Fat: 0g

SPICY PICKLED BEANS

VEGAN | DAIRY-FREE | GRAIN-FREE | GLUTEN-FREE | NUT-FREE | SOY-FREE |
KID FRIENDLY | LOW-FODMAP

If you like a little kick in your beans, then this recipe is for you. Add these spicy beans to stir-fries and salads for a boost of flavor, or simply snack on them as is.

MAKES 1 QUART

Prep time: 10 minutes
Fermentation time: 2 weeks

½ pound young snap beans, trimmed

1 teaspoon whole black peppercorns

3 fresh serrano chiles, stemmed and seeded, sliced lengthwise into thin strips

2 tablespoons pickling salt

3 cups water

Phase 2 Tip: Add 2 to 4 cloves of crushed garlic to the jar in step 1.

1. Layer the beans, peppercorns, and chile strips in a quart jar.

2. In a small bowl, combine the pickling salt and water, stirring until the salt is completely dissolved. Pour the brine over the beans. Use a small weight to hold the beans below the surface (see page 242). Cover with a lid, airlock, or bag filled with any remaining brine (see page 245), and set aside at room temperature.

3. Within a few days, bubbles will begin rising to the surface. Check the jar daily for scum on the surface. If any forms, use a nonreactive spoon to remove it promptly, then rinse the weight and return it to the jar.

4. In about 2 weeks fermentation will be complete, and bubbles will stop rising to the surface. Remove the weight, seal with the lid, and refrigerate for up to 3 months.

PER SERVING: (1/2 cup) Calories: 11, Protein: <1g, Cholesterol: 0mg, Sodium: 363mg, Total Carbohydrates: 3g, Fiber: 1g, Total Fat: <1g, Saturated Fat: 0g

KEFIR

VEGETARIAN | GRAIN-FREE | GLUTEN-FREE | NUT-FREE | SOY-FREE |
KID-FRIENDLY | LOW-FODMAP

Kefir is a probiotic powerhouse, and, when you make it yourself, it is very cost effective. Requiring minimal work, kefir is a room-temperature dairy ferment, making it about the simplest of them all. This recipe can be scaled up to 1 quart of kefir per day if you find yourself going through more than a pint daily.

MAKES 1 PINT

Prep time: 10 minutes
Fermentation time: 12 to 24 hours

1 tablespoon kefir grains (if starting with dehydrated kefir grains, see sidebar on following page)
2 cups whole milk

1. Add the kefir grains to a pint jar. Pour in the milk.

2. Cover the jar using a clean cloth or nonreactive lid loosely applied. Set aside at room temperature for 12 to 24 hours, until thickened.

3. Strain the grains from the kefir using a nonreactive strainer placed over another pint jar; reserve the grains.

4. Seal the jar with a lid and refrigerate for up to 5 days.

5. Place the reserved grains in a new pint jar, fill with milk, and begin the process again.

PER SERVING: (1/4 cup) Calories: 31, Protein: 2g, Cholesterol: 5mg, Sodium: 29mg, Total Carbohydrates: 3g, Fiber: 0g, Total Fat: 1g Saturated Fat: <1g,

REHYDRATING KEFIR GRAINS

If starting with dehydrated (instead of ready-to-go) kefir grains, be sure follow this procedure to rehydrate them before starting the recipe.

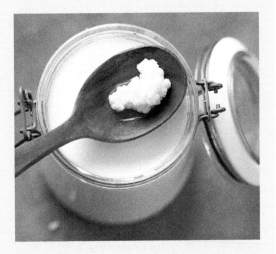

To get started with kefir making, you will need to purchase kefir grains, which typically are shipped in a dehydrated state. To rehydrate the grains, place them in 1 cup of cold milk, and cover the jar with a clean kitchen towel secured with a rubber band. After 24 hours, strain the grains from the milk and add them to a fresh cup of milk (discard the strained milk). Continue this process until the milk thickens within a 24-hour period. When it thickens, increase the milk to 1½ cups until it thickens within a 24-hour period, at which time you add 2 cups of milk. You can continue with this process until you have 4 cups of milk, or stop at 2 cups and make just 1 pint of kefir daily. As long as you keep feeding the kefir grains with new milk, you can keep reusing the grains indefinitely. Once you stop using them, they will die and need to be discarded.

CINNAMON-PEACH KEFIR

VEGETARIAN | GRAIN-FREE | GLUTEN-FREE | NUT-FREE | SOY-FREE |
KID-FRIENDLY | LOW-FODMAP

Once you master making plain kefir, don't stop there. You can second ferment your kefir using any number of flavorings to create an even tastier end product that has even higher levels of B vitamins. An additional day on the counter, paired with fresh or frozen fruits, increases flavor, creates a fizzy beverage, and it becomes even creamier. Be sure to strain the kefir grains and start a new batch in another jar before beginning a second ferment.

MAKES 1 QUART

Prep time: 10 minutes
Fermentation time: 12 to 24 hours

---

2 cups plain milk kefir
2 cups puréed peaches
1 cinnamon stick

Variation Tip: Try making second ferments with any fruits you like using a similar ratio. You can also use garlic (in Phase 2), herbs, spices, and extracts in kefir for different flavors.

In a quart jar, combine the kefir, peaches, and cinnamon. Cover with the lid and set aside at room temperature for 12 to 24 hours until thickened. Discard the cinnamon stick. Refrigerate for 1 hour to chill before serving. The kefir will keep in an airtight container at room temperature for up to 5 days.

PER SERVING: (1/4 cup) Calories: 47, Protein: 2g, Cholesterol: 5mg, Sodium: 116mg, Total Carbohydrates: 7g, Fiber: <1g, Total Fat: 1g, Saturated Fat: <1g

YOGURT

VEGETARIAN | GRAIN-FREE | GLUTEN-FREE | NUT-FREE | SOY-FREE |
KID-FRIENDLY | LOW-FODMAP

Yogurt is slightly more hands-on than kefir making, but you are rewarded for your hard work. Homemade yogurt is creamy and rich, and has a delicious sweetness. It is important that the ferment be maintained at a higher temperature, about 110°F, during fermentation, making it necessary to use equipment. Many food dehydrators have a setting for this, or you can use an insulated cooler or lunchbox with great results. For the yogurt starter, purchase a plain, unsweetened, full-fat yogurt that has active cultures present; read the label and select one without added fillers, such as gelatin or dried milk powder. Be sure to reserve ¼ cup of yogurt from each batch so you can continue making yogurt without having to buy new starter every time.

MAKES 1 QUART

Prep time: 5 minutes
Cook time: 5 minutes
Fermentation time: 12 to 24 hours

3¾ cups whole milk
¼ cup yogurt starter

1. In a saucepan, heat the milk until it reaches 180°F. Immediately remove the pan from the heat and let the milk cool to 110°F. To expedite the process, immerse the bottom of the pot in an ice bath.

2. Pour the yogurt starter into a clean quart jar. Pour the warmed milk into the jar, leaving 1 inch of headspace at the top. Cover the jar with the lid and shake to combine.

3. Place the jar in your chosen insulated incubator. If you are using an insulated lunchbox, fill a jar with hot water, place it next to the yogurt jar in the lunchbox, and close the lunchbox. If you are using a cooler with ridged sides, fill the cooler with hot water up to the neck of the jar. Close the incubator.

4. Yogurt takes 12 to 24 hours to ferment. Depending on the length of time and your incubator, you may need to refresh the hot water to maintain a temperature above 110°F in the incubator. Check the yogurt after 12 hours. If it is not adequately thickened, ferment it for up to 24 hours. When done, refrigerate for up to 5 days.

PER SERVING: (1/2 cup) Calories: 87, Protein: 7g, Cholesterol: 7mg, Sodium: 86mg, Total Carbohydrates: 9g, Fiber: 0g, Total Fat: 2g, Saturated Fat: 1g

Phase 2 Tip: For a nutritional boost in Phase 2, top your yogurt with blueberries, mint, and a generous drizzle of raw honey.

SPICED LASSI

VEGETARIAN | GRAIN-FREE | GLUTEN-FREE | SOY-FREE | KID FRIENDLY | LOW-FODMAP

Spiced lassis may not be a mainstay in America (yet), but in India, the birthplace of the lassi, this type of simple yogurt drink is a typical digestive tonic used regularly to maintain health. Loaded with warming ginger, nutmeg, and cardamom, this savory drink is filling and soothing.

MAKES 1 DRINK

Prep time: 5 minutes

---

1 cup plain yogurt (not fat-free)
2 tablespoons unsweetened almond milk or coconut milk
1 tablespoon pure maple syrup
1 teaspoon ground ginger
½ teaspoon ground nutmeg
½ teaspoon ground cardamom
Fresh mint leaves, for garnish

Variation Tip: Maple syrup is added here to give the drink a slight sweetness. You can omit it for a more sour, yet still delicious and well-seasoned drink. For a more minty version of the beverage, add 1 tablespoon of freshly chopped mint in step 1, and garnish with the mint leaves, too.

1. In a blender, combine the yogurt, milk, maple syrup, ginger, nutmeg, and cardamom and blend until well combined.

2. Pour into a small glass and serve garnished with torn mint leaves.

PER SERVING: Calories: 311, Protein: 15g, Cholesterol: 15mg, Sodium: 179mg, Total Carbohydrates: 35g, Fiber: 1g, Total Fat: 11g, Saturated Fat: 9g

MANGO LASSI

VEGETARIAN | GRAIN-FREE | GLUTEN-FREE | NUT-FREE | SOY-FREE |
KID FRIENDLY | LOW-FODMAP

Mango lassi, made popular by the large Indian diaspora around the world, is a refreshing drink on a hot day. The sweetness of the mango shines in this simple fermented beverage. If you are not making your own yogurt (page 258), be sure to select one that has live cultures in it for maximum benefit.

MAKES 2 DRINKS

Prep time: 10 minutes

1 cup frozen mango
1 cup plain yogurt (not fat-free)
1 teaspoon confectioners' sugar
Fresh mint leaves, for garnish

Ingredient Tip: The price on mangos can vary a lot throughout the year. Next time you see them on sale, pick up a few extra. You can peel, stone, and chop them into cubes to freeze and use later.

1. In a blender, combine the mango, yogurt, and confectioners' sugar and blend until smooth.

2. Divide evenly between 2 glasses. Garnish with mint and serve.

PER SERVING: Calories: 92, Protein: 7g, Cholesterol: 7mg, Sodium: 287mg, Total Carbohydrates: 10g, Fiber: 0g, Total Fat: 2g, Saturated Fat: 1g

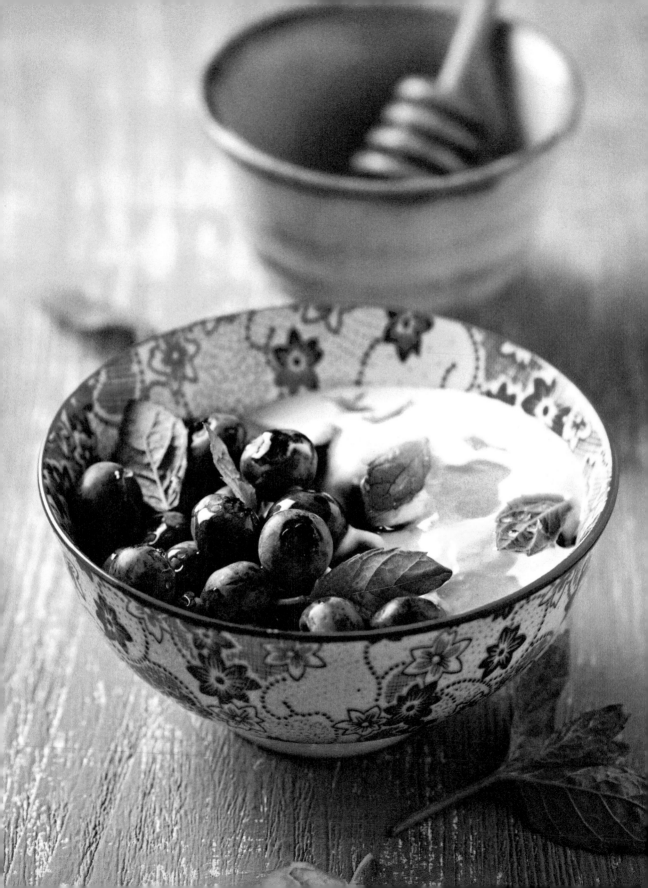

THE DIRTY DOZEN & THE CLEAN FIFTEEN

A nonprofit and environmental watchdog organization called Environmental Working Group (EWG) looks at data supplied by the US Department of Agriculture (USDA) and the Food and Drug Administration (FDA) about pesticide residues. Each year it compiles a list of the best and worst pesticide loads found in commercial crops. You can use these lists to decide which fruits and vegetables to buy organic to minimize your exposure to pesticides and which produce is considered safe enough to buy conventionally. This does not mean they are pesticide-free, though, so wash these fruits and vegetables thoroughly.

These lists change every year, so make sure you look up the most recent one before you fill your shopping cart. You'll find the most recent lists as well as a guide to pesticides in produce at EWG.org/FoodNews.

2016 Dirty Dozen

Apples	Nectarines	*In addition to the dirty dozen, the EWG added two produce contaminated with highly toxic organo-phosphate insecticides:*
Celery	Peaches	
Cherries	Spinach	
Cherry Tomatoes	Strawberries	
Cucumbers	Sweet bell peppers	Kale/Collard greens
Grapes	Tomatoes	Hot peppers

2016 Clean Fifteen

Asparagus	Corn	Mangos
Avocados	Eggplant	Onions
Cabbage	Grapefruit	Papayas
Cantaloupe	Honeydew Melon	Pineapple
Cauliflower	Kiwi	Sweet Peas (frozen)

CONVERSION TABLES

Volume Equivalents (Liquid)

US STANDARD	US STANDARD (OUNCES)	METRIC (APPROXIMATE)
2 tablespoons	1 fl. oz.	30 mL
¼ cup	2 fl. oz.	60 mL
½ cup	4 fl. oz.	120 mL
1 cup	8 fl. oz.	240 mL
1½ cups	12 fl. oz.	355 mL
2 cups or 1 pint	16 fl. oz.	475 mL
4 cups or 1 quart	32 fl. oz.	1 L
1 gallon	128 fl. oz.	4 L

Oven Temperatures

FAHRENHEIT (F)	CELSIUS (C) (APPROXIMATE)
250°	120°
300°	150°
325°	165°
350°	180°
375°	190°
400°	200°
425°	220°
450°	230°

Volume Equivalents (Dry)

US STANDARD	METRIC (APPROXIMATE)
⅛ teaspoon	0.5 mL
¼ teaspoon	1 mL
½ teaspoon	2 mL
¾ teaspoon	4 mL
1 teaspoon	5 mL
1 tablespoon	15 mL
¼ cup	59 mL
⅓ cup	79 mL
½ cup	118 mL
⅔ cup	156 mL
¾ cup	177 mL
1 cup	235 mL
2 cups or 1 pint	475 mL
3 cups	700 mL
4 cups or 1 quart	1 L

Weight Equivalents

US STANDARD	METRIC (APPROXIMATE)
½ ounce	15 g
1 ounce	30 g
2 ounces	60 g
4 ounces	115 g
8 ounces	225 g
12 ounces	340 g
16 ounces or 1 pound	455 g

RESOURCES

If you search online for information about the microbiome, you'll come across many websites that misleadingly interpret the science and connect illegitimate dots. The following is a list of credible resources on the role of the microbiome in health.

Microbiome & Diet Resources

Gut Microbiota for Health
gutmicrobiotaforhealth.com/en
/home

International Scientific Association for Probiotics and Prebiotics (ISAPP)
isappscience.org

The Intestinal Gardener Blog
intestinalgardener.blogspot.com

ISAPP Clinical Guide to Probiotic Supplements in Canada
probioticchart.ca

ISAPP Clinical Guide to Probiotic Products in the United States
usprobioticguide.com

Microbiome News
news.microbiomeproject.com

Monash University Low FODMAP Diet App
med.monash.edu/cecs/gastro
/fodmap/iphone-app.html

Monash University Low FODMAP Diet for Irritable Bowel Syndrome
med.monash.edu/cecs/gastro
/fodmap

Translational Microbiome Research Forum
translationalmicrobiome.org

University of Massachusetts Medical School IBD-AID Diet
umassmed.edu/nutrition/ibd/ibdaid

Microbiome Books

Blaser, M. J. *Missing Microbes: How the Overuse of Antibiotics Is Fueling Our Modern Plagues.* New York: Henry Holt and Co., 2014.

Collen, A. *10% Human: How Your Body's Microbes Hold the Key to Health and Happiness.* New York: HarperCollins, 2015.

Knight, R., and B. Buhler. *Follow Your Gut: The Enormous Impact of Tiny Microbes.* New York: Simon & Schuster, 2015.

Sonnenburg, J., and E. Sonnenburg. *The Good Gut: Taking Control of Your Weight, Your Mood, and Your Long-Term Health.* New York: Penguin Press, 2015.

Microbiome Research Participation

American Gut
americangut.org

National Institutes of Health
Clinical Studies Database
clinicaltrials.gov

Fermentation Supplies & Resources

Cultures for Health
culturesforhealth.com

Fermenters Club
fermentersclub.com

Wild Fermentation Facebook Group
facebook.com/groups
/WlidFermentation/

Katz, S. E. *The Art of Fermentation: An In-Depth Exploration of Essential Concepts and Processes from Around the World.* White River Junction: Chelsea Green, 2012.

Katz, S. E. *Wild Fermentation: The Flavor, Nutrition, and Craft of Live-Culture Foods.* White River Junction: Chelsea Green, 2003.

NOTES

Chapter One

1. Marchesi, J. R. & J. Ravel. "The Vocabulary of Microbiome Research: a Proposal." *Microbiome* 3, no. 31 (July 2015). doi:10.1186/s40168-015-0094-5.

2. Zhang, X., D. Zhang, H. Jia, et al. "The Oral and Gut Microbiomes Are Perturbed in Rheumatoid Arthritis and Partly Normalized after Treatment." *Nature Medicine* 21 (July 2015): 895–905. doi:10.1038/nm.3914.

3. da Fonseca D. M., T. W. Hand, et al. "Microbiota-Dependent Sequelae of Acute Infection Compromise Tissue-Specific Immunity." *Cell* 63, no. 2 (October 2015): 354–66. doi:10.1016/j.cell.2015.08.030.

4. Alcock, J., C. C. Maley & C. A. Aktipis. "Is Eating Behavior Manipulated by the Gastrointestinal Microbiota? Evolutionary Pressures and Potential Mechanisms." *BioEssays* 36, no. 10 (2014): 940–949. doi:10.1002/bies.201400071.

5. Breton, J., et al. "Gut Commensal E. coli Proteins Activate Host Satiety Pathways following Nutrient-Induced Bacterial Growth." *Cell Metabolism* 23, no. 2 (February 2016): 1–11.

6. Tillisch, K., et al. "Consumption of Fermented Milk Product with Probiotic Modulates Brain Activity." *Gastroenterology* 144, no. 7 (June 2013). doi:10.1053/j.gastro.2013.02.043.

7. Messaoudi, M., et al. "Assessment of Psychotropic-Like Properties of a Probiotic Formulation (*Lactobacillus helveticus* R0052 and *Bifidobacterium longum* R0175) in Rats and Human Subjects." *British Journal of Nutrition* 105, no. 5 (2011): 755–64. doi: http://dx.doi.org/10.1017/S0007114510004319.

8. Hilimire, M. R., et al. "Fermented Foods, Neuroticism, and Social Anxiety: An Interaction Model." *Psychiatry Research* 228, no. 2 (August 2015): 203–208. doi:10.1016/j.psychres.2015.04.023.

9. Jiang, H., et al. "Altered Fecal Microbiota Composition in Patients with Major Depressive Disorder." *Brain, Behavior, and Immunity* 48 (August 2015): 186–94. doi:10.1016/j.bbi.2015.03.016.

10. Bercik, P., et al. "The Intestinal Microbiota Affect Central Levels of Brain-Derived Neurotropic Factor and Behavior in Mice." *Gastroenterology* 141, no. 2 (August 2011): 599–609. doi: http://dx.doi.org/10.1053/j.gastro.2011.04.052.

11. Christian, L. M., et al. "Gut Microbiome Composition Is Associated with Temperament during Early Childhood." *Brain, Behavior, and Immunity* 45, Issue Null (November 2014): 118–127. doi:10.1016/j.bbi.2014.10.018.

12. Kau, A. L., et al. "Human Nutrition, the Gut Microbiome, and Immune System: Envisioning the Future." *Nature* 474, no. 7,351 (June 2011): 327–36. doi:10.1038/nature10213.

13. Hehemann, J.-H., et al. "Bacteria of the Human Gut Microbiome Catabolize Red Seaweed Glycans with Carbohydrate-Active Enzyme Updates from Extrinsic Microbes." *Proceedings of the National Academy of Sciences of the United States of America* 109, no. 48 (November 2012): 19786–91 doi:10.1073/pnas.1211002109.

14. Sanders, Mary Ellen. "Probiotics." International Scientific Association for Probiotics and Prebiotics. Accessed April 14, 2016. isappscience.org/probiotics.

Chapter Two

15. Zeevi, D., et al. "Personalized Nutrition by Prediction of Glycemic Responses." *Cell* 163, no. 5 (November 2015): 1079–94. doi: http://dx.doi.org/10.1016/j.cell.2015.11.001.

16. Marsh, A., E. M. Eslick & G. D. Eslick. "Does a Diet Low in FODMAPs Reduce Symptoms Associated with Functional Gastrointestinal Disorders? A Comprehensive Systematic Review and Meta-Analysis." *European Journal of Nutrition* 55, no. 3 (April 2016): 897–906. doi:10.1007/s00394-015-0922-1.

17. Charlebois, A., G. Rosenfeld & B. Bressler. "The Impact of Dietary Interventions on the Symptoms of Inflammatory Bowel Disease: A Systematic Review." *Critical Reviews in Food Science and Nutrition* (January 2015): e-pub ahead of print. doi:10.1080/10408398.2012.760515

18. Halmos, E. P., C. T. Christophersen, A. R. Bird, S. J. Shepherd, P. R. Gibson & J. G. Muir. "Diets that Differ in Their FODMAP Content Alter the Colonic Luminal Microenvironment." *Gut* 64, no. 1 (January 2015): 93–100. doi:10.1136/gutjnl-2014-307264.

19. Olendzki, B.C., et al. "An Anti-Inflammatory Diet as Treatment for Inflammatory Bowel Disease: A Case Series Report." *Nutrition Journal* 13, no. 5 (January 2014): doi:10.1186/1475-2891-13-5.

20. Hehemann, J.-H., et al. "Bacteria of the Human Gut Microbiome Catabolize Red Seaweed Glycans with Carbohydrate-Active Enzyme Updates from Extrinsic Microbes." *Proceedings of the National Academy of Sciences of the United States of America* 109, no. 48 (November 2012): 19786–91. doi:10.1073/pnas.1211002109.

BIBLIOGRAPHY

Alcock, J., C. C. Maley & C. A. Aktipis. "Is Eating Behavior Manipulated by the Gastrointestinal Microbiota? Evolutionary Pressures and Potential Mechanisms." *BioEssays* 36, no. 10 (2014): 940–949. doi:10.1002/bies.201400071.

Bercik, P., et al. "The Intestinal Microbiota Affect Central Levels of Brain-Derived Neurotropic Factor and Behavior in Mice." *Gastroenterology* 141, no. 2 (August 2011): 599–609. doi: http://dx.doi.org/10.1053/j .gastro.2011.04.052.

Breton, J., et al. "Gut Commensal *E. coli* Proteins Activate Host Satiety Pathways following Nutrient-Induced Bacterial Growth." *Cell Metabolism* 23, no. 2 (February 2016): 1–11.

Charlebois, A., G. Rosenfeld & B. Bressler. "The Impact of Dietary Interventions on the Symptoms of Inflammatory Bowel Disease: A Systematic Review." *Critical Reviews in Food Science and Nutrition* (January 2015): e-pub ahead of print. doi: 10.1080/10408398.2012.760515.

Christian, L. M., et al. "Gut Microbiome Composition Is Associated with Temperament during Early Childhood." *Brain, Behavior, and Immunity* 45, Issue Null (November 2014): 118–127. doi:10.1016/j. bbi.2014.10.018.

Chutkan, Robynne. *The Microbiome Solution: A Radical New Way to Heal Your Body from the Inside Out*. New York: Avery, 2015.

Cook's Illustrated Editors. *The New Best Recipe*. Boston: America's Test Kitchen, 2004.

da Fonseca D. M., T. W. Hand, et al. "Microbiota-Dependent Sequelae of Acute Infection Compromise Tissue-Specific Immunity." *Cell* 63, no.2 (October 2015): 354–66. doi:10.1016/j.cell.2015.08.030.

De Filippis F., et al. "High-Level Adherence to a Mediterranean Diet Beneficially Impacts the Gut Microbiota and Associated Metabolome." *Gut* (September 2015): doi:10.1136/gutjnl-2015-309957.

Dragonwagon, Crescent. *Soup & Bread: A Country Inn Cookbook*. New York: Workman Publishing Company, 1992.

Food and Agriculture Organization of the United Nations & World Health Organization. "Health and Nutritional Properties of Probiotics in Food Including Powder Milk with Live Lactic Acid Bacteria." Accessed February 2, 2016. ftp://ftp.fao .org/es/esn/food/probio_report_en.pdf.

Gut Microbiota for Health Research & Practice. "Messages about Diet and IBD Need to Change, says Canadian Researcher." Accessed February 17, 2016. gutmicrobiotaforhealth.com/en /messages-about-diet-and-ibd-need-to -change-says-canadian-researcher.

Graham, T. G. & D. Ramsey. *The Happiness Diet: A Nutritional Prescription for a Sharp Brain, Balanced Mood, and Lean, Energized Body.* New York: Rodale, 2011.

Halmos, E. P., C. T. Christophersen, A. R. Bird, S. J. Shepherd, P. R. Gibson & J. G. Muir. "Diets That Differ in Their FODMAP Content Alter the Colonic Luminal Microenvironment." *Gut* 64, no. 1 (January 2015): 93–100. doi:10.1136 /gutjnl-2014-307264.

Hawkes, Alex D. *Cooking with Vegetables.* New York: Simon & Schuster, 1968.

Hehemann, J.-H., et al. "Bacteria of the Human Gut Microbiome Catabolize Red Seaweed Glycans with Carbohydrate-Active Enzyme Updates from Extrinsic Microbes." *Proceedings of the National Academy of Sciences of the United States of America* 109, no. 48 (November 2012): 19786–91. doi:10.1073/pnas.1211002109.

Hilimire, M. R., et al. "Fermented Foods, Neuroticism, and Social Anxiety: An Interaction Model." *Psychiatry Research* 228, no. 2 (August 2015): 203–208. doi:10.1016/j.psychres.2015.04.023.

Iyer, Raghavan. *660 Curries.* New York: Workman Publishing Company, 2008.

Jiang, H., et al. "Altered Fecal Microbiota Composition in Patients with Major Depressive Disorder." *Brain, Behavior, and Immunity* 48 (August 2015): 186–94. doi:10.1016/j.bbi.2015.03.016.

Kau, A. L., et al. "Human Nutrition, the Gut Microbiome, and Immune System: Envisioning the Future." *Nature* 474, no. 7,351 (June 2011): 327–36. doi:10.1038/nature10213.

Kellman, Raphael. *The Microbiome Diet: The Scientifically Proven Way to Restore Your Gut Health and Achieve Permanent Weight Loss.* Boston: Da Capo Press, 2014.

Kobayashi, Katsuyo. *The Quick and Easy Japanese Cookbook.* New York: Kondansha America, Inc., 2000.

Koeth, R. A., et al. (2013) "Intestinal Microbiota Metabolism of L-carnitine, a Nutrient in Red Meat, Promotes Atherosclerosis." *Nature Medicine* 19, no. 5 (May 2013): 576–85. doi:10.1038 /nm.3145.

Marchesi, J. R. & J. Ravel. "The Vocabulary of Microbiome Research: a Proposal." *Microbiome* 3, no. 31 (July 2015). doi:10.1186/s40168-015-0094-5.

Marsh, A., E. M. Eslick & G. D. Eslick. "Does a Diet Low in FODMAPs Reduce Symptoms Associated with Functional Gastrointestinal Disorders? A Comprehensive Systematic Review and Meta-Analysis." *European Journal of Nutrition* 55, no. 3 (April 2016): 897–906. doi:10.1007/s00394-015-0922-1.

Messaoudi, M., et al. "Assessment of Psychotropic-Like Properties of a Probiotic Formulation (*Lactobacillus helveticus* R0052 and *Bifidobacterium longum* R0175) in Rats and Human Subjects." *British Journal of Nutrition* 105, no. 5 (2011): 755–64. doi: http://dx.doi.org/10.1017/S0007114510004319.

Monash University Medicine, Nursing, and Health Sciences. "The Monash University Low FODMAP Diet." Accessed February 17, 2016. med.monash.edu/cecs/gastro/fodmap/low-high.html.

Mozaffarian, D., et al. "Changes in Diet and Lifestyle and Long-Term Weight Gain in Women and Men." *New England Journal of Medicine* 364 (June 2011): 2392–2404. doi:10.1056/NEJMoa1014296.

Mullin, Gerard E. *The Gut Balance Revolution: Boost Your Metabolism, Restore Your Inner Ecology, and Lose the Weight for Good.* New York: Rodale, 2015.

Null, Gary & Shelly Null. *Vegetarian Cooking for Good Health.* New York: Collier Books, 1991.

Olendzki, B.C., et al. "An Anti-Inflammatory Diet as Treatment for Inflammatory Bowel Disease: A Case Series Report." *Nutrition Journal* 13, no. 5 (January 2014). doi:10.1186/1475-2891-13-5.

Practical Soups. Bath, UK: P³ Publishing, 2002.

Ridaura, V. K., et al. "Gut Microbiota from Twins Discordant for Obesity Modulate Metabolism in Mice." *Science* 341, no. 6,150 (September 2013). doi:10.1126/science.1241214.

Sanders, Mary Ellen. "Probiotics." International Scientific Association for Probiotics and Prebiotics. Accessed April 14, 2016. isappscience.org/probiotics.

Slavin, J. L. "Dietary Fiber and Body Weight." *Nutrition* 21, no. 3 (March 2005): 411–18. doi: http://dx.doi.org/10.1016/j.nut.2004.08.018.

Sonnenburg, Justin, and Sonnenburg, Erica. *The Good Gut: Taking Control of Your Weight, Your Mood, and Your Long-Term Health.* New York: Penguin Press, 2015.

Stulberg, E., et al. "An Assessment of US Microbiome Research." *Nature Microbiology* 1 (2016): 15015. doi:10.1038/nmicrobiol.2015.15.

Tillisch, K., et al. "Consumption of Fermented Milk Product with Probiotic Modulates Brain Activity." *Gastroenterology* 144, no. 7 (June 2013). doi:10.1053/j.gastro.2013.02.043.

University of Massachusetts Medical School Center for Applied Nutrition. "IBD-AID Diet." Accessed February 17, 2016. umassmed.edu/nutrition/ibd/ibdaid.

Wood, Rebecca. *The New Whole Foods Encyclopedia.* New York: Penguin Books, 2010.

Zeevi, D., et al. "Personalized Nutrition by Prediction of Glycemic Responses." *Cell* 163, no. 5 (November 2015): 1079–94. doi: http://dx.doi.org/10.1016/j.cell.2015.11.001.

Zhang, X., D. Zhang, H. Jia, et al. "The Oral and Gut Microbiomes Are Perturbed in Rheumatoid Arthritis and Partly Normalized after Treatment." *Nature Medicine* 21 (July 2015): 895–905. doi:10.1038/nm.3914.

Ziedrich, Linda. *The Joy of Pickling*. Boston: The Harvard Common Press, 1998.

RECIPE INDEX

INDEX

ABOUT THE AUTHOR

Science writer **KRISTINA CAMPBELL** specializes in communication about the gut microbiota. As a member of the Gut Microbiota for Health publishing team, she has interviewed dozens of experts on nutrition and the microbiome. She is a member of the Canadian Science Writers Association and an active freelance writer whose work has appeared in publications around the world, from Canada to Australia, and translated into French and Spanish. Kristina is co-author of an upcoming academic textbook on nutrition and gut microbiota.

Additional Resources for the Two Phases of the Microbiome Diet

PHASE ONE : REPAIR

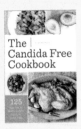

Candida Free
Sondi Bruner

Fight the overgrowth of Candida albicans, a yeast-like fungus that proliferates with unhealthy gut flora.

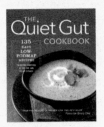

The Quiet Gut Cookbook
Sonoma Press

Enjoy 135 low-FODMAP recipes that can also be made free of common allergens like eggs, dairy, and shellfish.

PHASE TWO : RECOVERY

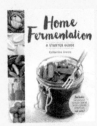

Home Fermentation
Katherine Green

Diversify your gut microbes with easy fermentation recipes for probiotic-packed foods and drinks.

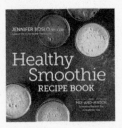

Healthy Smoothie Recipe Book
Jennifer Koslo

Customize and prepare nutrient-rich smoothies to feed your microbiome when you're on the go or too busy to cook.

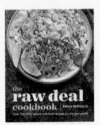

The Raw Deal Cookbook
Emily Monaco

Nourish your good gut flora by swapping starchy refined carbs with fiber-rich fruits and vegetables.

CPSIA information can be obtained
at www.ICGtesting.com
Printed in the USA
LVOW05s1721240916

505802LV00014B/14/P